TRY FOR DRY

A commonsense approach
to the problems of
Incontinence

By

Mary Medill

Published by Care Taker Ltd.
The Mead House,
Sherborne,
Glos. GL54 3DR

VAT Number: 535 622 55

Second Edition 1990
Third Edition 1991
Fourth Edition 1993

ISBN 0 9515701 3 7 ✓

Contents

ACKNOWLEDGEMENTS

I am grateful to:

Mr. Martin Claridge, MCH, FRCS, Consultant Urologist at the Kent and Canterbury Hospital, for giving great support, providing medical details and allowing me to pick his brains,

Dr. Jonathan Potter, MD, MRCP, Consultant Physician in Geriatric Medicine at the Kent and Canterbury Hospital, for expert comment and advice and for kindly writing the foreword,

Mr. David Sells, MA, for patient editing,

My husband, for much help and encouragement.

1989

I should like to thank also the Staffs of the Association for Continence Advice, the Dene Centre and the Continence Foundation for all the constructive help they have given me over the years. I am grateful also for all the help I have received from those doctors, continence advisers, physiotherapists and nurses whose lectures I have heard, whose papers and books I have read and who have answered many telephone queries.

1993   MARY MEDILL

Incontinence remains one of the commonest hidden disabilities, especially for the elderly, causing not only physical inconvenience and hardship but also psychological turmoil. Mary Medill's concise and sensible book *Try for Dry* is a welcome source of help.

The physiological and medical review explains in simple terms the various different ways in which incontinence can arise and indicates that this "problem" need not be a cause of despondency, but may well be treatable.

The practical guide to assessing and managing incontinence strikes a very positive note, and the optimism expressed in striving for continence is very welcome.

I am sure this production will provide a useful insight to sufferers and carers alike and help many achieve a better quality of life.

Dr Jonathan Potter, MD,MRCP,
Consultant Physician in Geriatric Medicine

INTRODUCTION

In the following pages there is much that is obvious and much that you will know already, because this book has been written for the whole range of sufferers, from the young to the very old. It is written also for those who care for them, whether relatives, friends or helpers. It is written in the hope of bringing something of value to every reader.

It is a little-known fact that nearly three million people in Britain suffer from problems of bladder control. This involuntary release of urine at any time is known as *urinary incontinence*. This is not in itself a disease, but a symptom of malfunction of the urinary system which may have a number of causes.

Naturally, the problem varies in severity, from a slight dampness resulting perhaps from coughing or sneezing, to a total loss of control. But for every person involved there is a feeling of embarrassment, discomfort and inconvenience; for others, more seriously affected, there is often a sense of inferiority and isolation.

One result of this is that incontinence is regarded as a *taboo* subject – something nobody talks about. In fact with this, as with all human problems, to share experience with a fellow-sufferer can be a great relief, especially when you realise what a common problem it is and how much can be done to help.

Continence is something we learn during the first two or three years of our life; it is a process of the bladder's telling the brain that it needs emptying, and the brain's replying with a message to the muscles controlling the bladder: either to hold on or to let go.

Incontinence is a sign that part of the system has gone wrong; we find it difficult to hold on. For some people it works the other way, and they find it difficult to let go.

In either case it is clear that something in your body is not working as it should and, as with any physical disorder, the first thing to do is to consult your doctor. Don't be embarrassed; to him, incontinence is as common and routine as a broken bone or measles – and much easier to cope with if treated early.

This book aims to help you with a particular problem by suggesting that you think methodically about your incontinence: by adopting slightly different habits, by doing certain exercises, and by keeping a chart of progress – at least to start with. These procedures have helped many people and *they can also help you*, so it is well worth taking them seriously.

Personal health is a central concern for any individual, but it is important to keep problems in perspective. On the one hand it is foolish to ignore simple health care but, on the other, if rules are followed too obsessively, one may end up with a fixation – perhaps about one's bladder or bowels.

So do remember that rules and methods are not an end in themselves; their purpose is simply to free you as far as possible from personal discomfort, and to enable you to live a fuller and happier life.

THE URINARY SYSTEM

On the opposite page there are two simple diagrams showing the urinary system in a woman and a man; the lower diagrams are on a larger scale, to show more detail.

A   Brain,

B   Part of the central nervous system, which runs through the spine and carries messages to and from the brain,

C   Kidneys,

D   Ureters, through which urine passes from the kidneys to the bladder,

E   Bladder,

F   Sphincter, the muscle controlling the outlet of the bladder,

G   Urethra, the tube through which urine is released,

H   Pelvic floor,

P   Prostate gland, only in men.

The kidneys act as filters which remove excess water, salts and waste products from the blood. This fluid, urine, trickles from the kidneys through two tubes called ureters into the bladder.

The bladder is a muscular bag which can stretch as urine collects; when the pressure increases, a message of discomfort is sent through the nerves to the brain. The brain replies with a message to:

1.   the muscles of the bladder,

2.   the sphincter, the muscle controlling the outlet of the bladder,

3.   the muscles of the floor of the pelvis.

The message is normally to hold on until you can reach a toilet, when the brain instructs the muscles of the bladder to contract and the sphincter to relax; this lets the urine out through the urethra.

In men, this tube is longer and includes the length of the penis. Another difference in men is the prostate gland, which lies below the bladder sphincter and above the pelvic floor and surrounds the urethra.

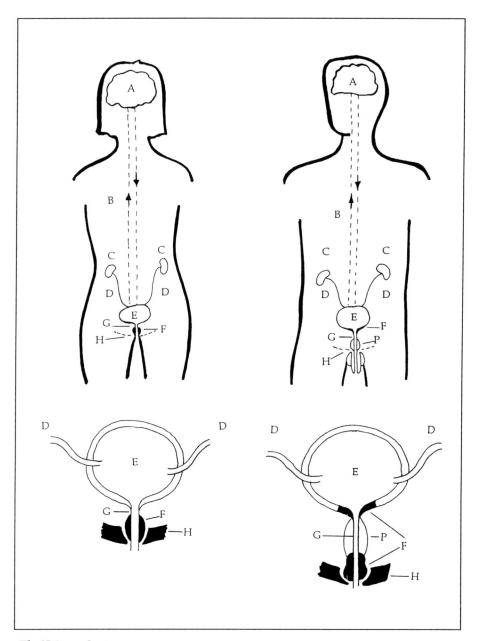

The Urinary System

As explained in the introduction, urinary incontinence varies greatly; it affects people of all ages, including the vigorous and active; there are various degrees of severity, and there are several different types and causes.

In order to describe these variations, incontinence is usually divided into five types, but these often overlap, so your particular case may well have elements of more than one type and more than one cause.

Don't be discouraged by thinking that your condition is bound to get worse. Just because you are incontinent as a young or middle-aged person, it does not mean that incontinence in old age is inevitable; much can be done.

Do go and see your doctor; many people suffer needlessly because they are too embarrassed to admit to incontinence, as though it were their fault. Many cases can be completely cured, and others can be greatly helped, but *your attitude is of vital importance*. You *must* be positive and determine to do everything you possibly can to minimise your incontinence and manage your problem; if you do this, you will gain peace of mind and the freedom to live as normally as possible.

STRESS

This word here refers to physical stress, not to a state of mind. Some people find that sudden movements, whether voluntary, such as lifting or bending, or convulsive, such as coughing or being sick, cause them to pass urine. This is known as Stress Incontinence.

Changes of body position, such as bending, and energetic or convulsive movements, such as lifting or coughing, which cause strong or sudden contraction of skeletal muscles, exert pressure on the bladder from outside; when this happens, the pressure inside the bladder rises and, unless the muscles of the pelvic floor and at the neck of the bladder are in good working order, they may be unable to contain the urine.

Weakness of the pelvic floor muscles is the main cause of this type of incontinence, and the commonest reason for this weakness is damage to the muscles from childbearing or surgery. Further contributory factors may be:

(a) physical structure; some women are more liable to this than others,

(b) additional bulk within the pelvis, as in early pregnancy, or constipation,

(c) irritation from infection in the bladder, from cystitis, and especially from prolapse of the uterus.

Women are the main sufferers from this type of incontinence and may need surgery. Men also are affected, sometimes after prostate operations. In all cases pelvic floor exercises are of great importance.

URGE

This is an overwhelming urgency to pass urine, resulting in not having enough time to get to the toilet before urinating. If this happens several times, a natural reaction is to start going to the toilet very often in order to forestall accidents. Unfortunately, this can make matters worse.

The most common cause is urinary infection, but it may be due to physical irritation from a variety of causes, for instance inflammation from some types of cystitis, bladder stones and oestrogen deficiency following the menopause.

Uncontrollable urgency happens also when the bladder is "unstable", a condition occurring when the "hold on" message from the brain is not strong enough to stop the bladder contracting.

Bladder instability occurs sometimes for no apparent reason; it may result from anxiety or confusion of mind, from diabetes or diseases of the nervous system. It may also occur after strokes or when the bladder is filled too rapidly after taking diuretics (water pills) or alcohol. The severity of the problem and the length of time it lasts vary widely; of course you should see your doctor. Bladder retraining schemes are effective for many sufferers.

Stress and Urge Incontinence are by far the commonest types; there are others.

OVERFLOW

This is a pattern of incontinence resulting from a bladder which cannot be emptied and remains full all the time. During the daytime, when the sufferer is awake, control can be exercised by frequent visits to the toilet,

15

although dribbling often occurs; at night water passes during sleep and results in bed-wetting. Men with prostatic obstruction often have this problem; it certainly should not be ignored, as ultimately the condition leads to back pressure on the kidneys and serious illness.

REFLEX

When there is an interruption of the spinal cord, as in spinal injury, messages cannot pass between the brain and the bladder, so normal control is partially or totally lost. As a result the bladder empties when it feels itself to be full, and the sufferer gets little or no sense of bladder fullness or of urinating. After a stroke, this interruption is due to damage to the part of the brain controlling the bladder.

Spinal trauma, diabetes, multiple sclerosis and some strokes are the main causes of reflex incontinence; it is not often realised that a slipped disc can cause incontinence, through pressure on the spinal nerves.

FUNCTIONAL

Incapacity of quite a different kind may make visits to the toilet difficult or impossible, so that incontinence results, even though the urinary tract is working properly. In some cases, such as accidents involving plaster casts or the period after an operation, this may be only a temporary condition, but in many others it can be a long-term one.

Causes may include head injuries, arthritis, partial or total blindness, strokes affecting the speech centre, Parkinson's disease, Alzheimer's disease, confusion of mind; even just sitting inactive for long periods can produce the same result.

VERY SEVERE INCONTINENCE

This is nearly always associated with diseases or disabilities. In children the disease may be cerebral palsy, Down's syndrome, spina bifida, malformation of the urinary tract or a number of others. In adults spinal injury, strokes, multiple sclerosis, Parkinson's disease, Alzheimer's disease and confusion associated with old age are some of the main offenders.

In these cases incontinence is just one of the problems facing both sufferers and helpers. Everybody concerned with the treatment will be coping with the problems but, because these are so immediate, people may not have considered or be aware of everything that can be done for incontinence. Do contact your continence adviser and if there isn't one in your area, see the address of the Continence Advisers Association at the back of the book. Treatment may include medication, catheterisation, penile appliances or perhaps surgery; your doctor will be aware that there may be complications to surgery, such as infection, but the advantages may well outweigh this consideration. For example, there are now operations to re-construct bladders, and artificial sphincters* can be made. Help may be available also in the form of financial aid or support for helpers. More and more use is made of intermittent self-catheterisation; many quite young children manage this by themselves.

These are ingenious devices consisting of a fluid-filled system with a small reservoir implanted under the skin of the abdomen and connected by a tube with an inflatable collar round the urethra; this can be inflated to close the urethra and retain urine, or deflated to release it, by means of switches placed on either side of the base of the scrotum in men, and in a similar position for women.

INFECTIONS

The most common cause of temporary incontinence is an infection of the urine or of the urinary tract. This causes inflammation of the bladder and the urethra, making the bladder unstable. The symptoms are a burning feeling when passing water, urgency and frequency.

Incontinence may get worse, also you may have cloudy and very strong-smelling urine, a temperature and a back pain. Do go to your doctor at once.

In the meantime, although this may seem surprising when you are suffering from frequency, you should drink more water but avoid fizzy drinks, tea, coffee and alcohol. Infections can become chronic, so do follow your doctor's instructions. For example, young men may have serious problems with persistent dribbling if the infection is prolonged, and women with chronic low-grade infections may be incontinent without any other symptoms appearing.

The symptoms of cystitis are very like those of urinary infection and are almost always associated to some degree with it. It is more common in women than in men, and contributory causes are varied.

It is often called "bride's disease", as very frequent and energetic sexual intercourse often starts an attack. Do remember to urinate before and after sexual intercourse. Vaginal infections, such as thrush, and infections from bacteria normal in the bowel but giving trouble in the bladder may cause cystitis. Irritation from tight or damp clothing and biological washing powders are also factors. People who cannot empty their bladder completely, leaving a large residue of urine, are prone to this complaint, as are men with prostate trouble.

At the first sign of symptoms, drink at least a pint of water an hour and keep on drinking; a small amount of bicarbonate of soda in the water is helpful.

Consult your doctor as soon as you can; meanwhile wear loose clothing made of natural fibres and avoid detergents and scented soaps. Wiping yourself from front to back helps keep bowel bacteria away from the urinary opening; make sure that your bladder is as empty as possible after every toilet visit. These precautions will help to prevent the symptoms. Chronic cystitis may be almost without symptoms other than incontinence.

WOMEN'S PROBLEMS

CHILDBIRTH

Difficult or repeated births, and births where natural tearing occurs or surgical cutting is necessary, may cause permanent damage to the pelvic floor, leading to stress incontinence; the same may apply after surgery for prolapse and after some hysterectomies.

Pelvic floor exercises are of extreme importance and very effective; electrical treatment is given to re-educate and strengthen the muscles.

PROLAPSED UTERUS

When the uterus is prolapsed, it slips down through the main envelope of the abdomen; this means that there is no muscular support for it and, more important, little or none for the neck of the bladder. This causes pressure on the urethra and added strain on the pelvic floor. When there is a small prolapse, or cystocele, the urethra may become kinked. These factors add to the problems of continence and sometimes cause difficulty in voiding, or occasionally retention of urine. Rings can be used to support the uterus, but usually surgery is recommended. Pelvic floor exercises and electrical treatment can help.

Some women with stress incontinence find that it increases slightly before menstruation, so it is as well to be aware of this and take precautions if necessary.

When women use tampons, they sometimes find it difficult to empty their bladders completely, so there may be a leak while removing a tampon or after doing so.

During early pregnancy many women have increased frequency, those with stress incontinence finding it even worse; this is quite natural and it normally decreases as the foetus grows and moves.

After the menopause women lack oestrogen, and this has an effect on the vaginal and urethral walls and so contributes to incontinence; hormone replacement therapy is an option which your doctor may consider.

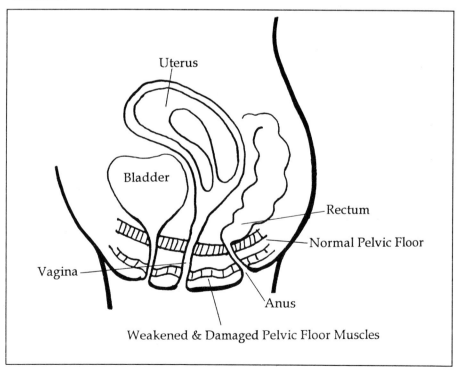

Strong and Weak Pelvic Floor Muscles

It is well known that, from middle age onwards, many men suffer from difficulty in urinating; not only are there difficulties in starting (i.e. "hesitancy") and a reduced stream, but there is also the problem of dribbling after the main stream has stopped.

These symptoms suggest that there has been some enlargement of the prostate gland, which surrounds the urethra below the bladder. Normally, when men have finished urinating, the urine contained in the urethra between the bladder neck and the pelvic floor "milks back" into the bladder; however, with the effects of age and an enlarged prostate, the mechanism does not work so well, and there will be a leak after the stream is finished. As the prostate enlarges further, urgency and frequency follow, many men having to get up four or five times a night. When the bladder contracts to expel urine, the muscle has to pull open the bladder neck; this is made more difficult by an enlarged prostate gland. The bladder has to work harder, and it takes longer to start expelling urine – this is "hesitancy". Consequently the bladder muscle gets thicker and stronger and relaxes less easily to accommodate urine, so producing frequency, urgency and instability. If urgency cannot be resisted, precipitancy, or even incontinence, may result.

In time the job of emptying becomes more difficult for the bladder muscle, and it begins to fail, leaving some urine behind. As this residual urine increases, the bladder muscle gets overstretched and consequently less efficient, which may result in:

(a)   a total inability to open the bladder neck and start urinating, which is known as "acute retention", or

(b)   such a large quantity of residual urine that the bladder is always full and empties only by overflowing, which is known as "chronic retention" or "overflow incontinence".

Go to your doctor when the symptoms appear; less damage will be done and results will therefore be better. This condition will need treatment by drugs and perhaps surgery. Meanwhile the following suggestions may be helpful.

1. When you have problems in starting a stream, try whistling, rustling paper or running a tap. If you are in pain, sitting in warm water often helps.

2. If your stream is diminished and stops and starts, try to relax and not to worry (perhaps easier said than done!) If you are dribbling, wait for a minute or two after finishing, and more urine will come; also, try going through the routine for emptying the bladder given on page 40.

3. Don't leave over-long intervals between visits to the toilet; it is when the bladder gets full that overflows occur.

4. Make out a Chart 1 and see how your drinking patterns affect your visits; then try to drink at times that will make life easier. But do drink enough, as this will help you to avoid constipation (see below). Eight to twelve cups a day is a guideline.

After a prostate operation:

1. Healing after an operation takes time; don't expect too much too soon.

2. Again, do remember to wait for a minute or so after your main stream finishes; there will *most probably* be more to come.

3. Do pelvic floor exercises regularly; they are important now (see page 32).

4. If you or your doctor think that your frequent visits to the toilet are due to habit, or that your bladder has become sensitive, try following the retraining routine for Group A1 on page 59.

5. Pants with rewashable built-in pads are practical and help you to avoid embarrassment.

6. Sometimes semen leaks back into the bladder after intercourse, and this may make the urine cloudy. It will pass in time and will not affect your bladder or your erection.

This is a very common problem. Men find that, especially as they approach middle age, in spite of waiting for a few moments and shaking the penis when finished, because some urine syphons back towards the bladder, a small leak appears several minutes later and often wets clothing.

This problem can be cured simply by applying forward pressure – about three fingers' width – behind the scrotum; this pushes the urine which has moved backwards towards the bladder down the penis again. To make sure, repeat the pressure a couple of times.

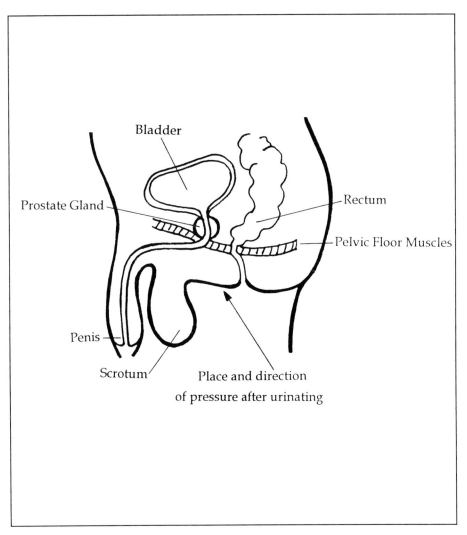

How to limit after-dribbles.

Many sufferers from incontinence do not drink enough, because they feel that drinking will increase their problem; however, not drinking can cause constipation, and this aggravates incontinence. A heavily loaded rectum not only occupies space within the pelvis and distorts the architecture of urinary outflow, but also, if there is unease in the rectum, this is felt as unease in the bladder.

It has been found that straining while at stool damages the muscles of the pelvic floor. Thus, even when young, constipation is not good for you. If faecal incontinence occurs, a weak pelvic floor is a contributory factor.

Do drink enough, eight to twelve cups a day; doing so is the best natural laxative. Eat sensibly, with plenty of what used to be called "roughage", high-fibre bread, cereals and plenty of green vegetables.

OTHER UNDERLYING CAUSES

There may be other underlying causes of your incontinence which your doctor will already know about or will be at pains to trace. Diabetes, for example, is a relatively common cause of incontinence; Parkinson's disease, endocrine disorders, anaemia, cardiac failure and anxiety are some of the others. All these can be treated by your doctor with marked success. This is why it is important to answer the questions on pages 24 and 25 to help him.

EFFECTS OF MEDICATION

Some medicines, taken for quite other reasons, can affect your continence, so make a note of what you are taking, to tell your doctor; for instance, sleeping pills may make you sleep through the need to urinate, and diuretics (water pills) can cause your bladder to fill too quickly and so make you incontinent. On the other hand, the doctor has a whole range of medicines that can relieve your symptoms.

Nearly all elderly people have a strong desire to remain continent; if medical help is sought in time, and the right conditions can be created, people who might have lapsed into incontinence can be treated and retain their independence.

In later life all reflexes slow down, and we take longer to react to circumstances; we become less aware of parts of our body, so accidental incontinence is more likely. Mobility is reduced to some extent for everyone, and for many almost entirely. Muscular tone is made worse by pain-killers and muscle relaxants. Balance is also affected, and elderly people have to take time before moving about after standing up. For men, the "milk-back" system of urine in the urethra become less efficient. Difficulties of communication may increase owing to deafness, blindness or the inability to speak. Of course, many elderly people do not suffer from incontinence at all, but any of the factors mentioned above, when combined with a disease such as diabetes, Parkinson's or anaemia, can gradually lead to a lesser or greater loss of continence. Once incontinence is established, morale and self-respect may be rapidly eroded, and the determination to be continent may be lost. Therefore it is *vitally* important to consult your doctor in good time, so that he can diagnose the underlying causes and arrange prompt treatment.

ATTITUDES

The mental attitude of each individual plays a vital part in the bodily functions and ageing process. Loneliness is a major cause of negative attitudes such as lethargy, boredom, depression and lack of self-respect, all of which contribute to a degeneration which may gradually slip into loss of control. Bereavement and anxiety also may cause incontinence. Alzheimer's disease or confusion of mind may result in toilet-training's being lost altogether.

QUESTIONS TO ASK YOURSELF WHICH WILL HELP YOUR DOCTOR'S DIAGNOSIS

If you are suddenly incontinent or have a feeling of burning, pain or illness, go to your doctor at once. Don't be tempted to try to diagnose the trouble yourself after reading the previous pages; there may well be other causes and aspects which your doctor will want to take into consideration.

However, if you have had this problem for a while, and it is not acute, you can help him by asking yourself the following simple questions about your symptoms and making a list of the answers over a period of two or three days. On the following page is Chart 1, which has been filled in as an example. You will find a blank chart at the back of the book, and it is most important that you fill it in on three consecutive days, not only for your doctor but also to provide information that will help you to correct or reduce your incontinence, as is described in the retraining programme on page 58.

When you go to the doctor, take your chart as well as the answers to the questions.

Most important: either take with you a sample of urine taken in mid-stream, or don't go to the toilet just before your visit, so that you are able to produce a sample if needed.

1.   Do you "leak" a little when you laugh, sneeze or cough?
2.   Or when you move suddenly, bend down or lift something?
3.   How long can you hold water after getting the urge to urinate?
4.   Do you have a constant or intermittent dribble?
5.   Do you urinate on the way to the toilet?
6.   How often do you get to the toilet in time? (For example, 2 out of 3 times).
7.   About how often do you get the urge?
8.   Does your bladder empty without warning?
9.   Do you feel that you are going to leak, or do you just find that you have leaked, without any sensation of doing so?
10.   Do you have to wait for a stream to start?
11.   Is the stream not as good as it was?
12.   Do you wake up wet?
13.   Does wetting wake you up?
14.   Are you taking any drugs? If so, which ones?
15.   Does it sting when you pass water?
16.   Do you often feel thirsty?
17.   How long does it take to get to the toilet?
18.   Do you have any difficulty in getting there?

You will no doubt have different routines for some days, but do fill in times for three consecutive days on the blank form at the back of the book, Chart 1. Put a tick (✔) for normal times of meals or snacks and put the number of cups of liquid you drink in the "amount" column. Then put a tick when applicable in the "urgency" column and a tick or cross in the "success" column, showing whether you managed to get to the toilet in time. In the "urine amount" column put the amount of urine in cups or fluid ounces. In the "medicine" column put type of medicine you have taken.

This first chart is filled in as an example.

Information for this chart can be recorded on the chart at the back of the book.

	meal	snack	drink (amount)	urgency	success	urine (amount)	medicine
Morning 7.00			1 cup	✓	✗	1 cup	general and diuretics
8.00				✓✓	✓✗	½ cup	
9.00	✓		1½ cups	✓	✓	½ cup	
10.00				✓	✗	1 cup	
11.00		✓	1 cup				
12.00				✓	✓	½ cup	
Afternoon 1.00		✓	1½ cups	✓	✓	½ cup	general
2.00							
3.00				✓	✗	½ cup	
4.00		✓	1½ cups				
5.00					✓	½ cup	
Evening 6.00							general and diuretics
7.00	✓		2 cups	✓	✓	1 cup	
8.00				✓✓✓	✓✗✓	1 cup	
9.00				✓✓	✓✓	½ cup	
10.00		✓	1 cup	✓✓	✗✓	½ cup	sleeping pill
Night 11.00							
12.00				✓	✗	1 cup	
1.00							
2.00							
3.00							
4.00				✓	✓	½ cup	
5.00							
6.00							
Total drunk and passed during day			9½ cups			9½ cups	

When you go to your doctor with the answers to your questions and your chart, he will most probably discuss your problems with you and examine you thoroughly. His aim will be to find out *why* you are incontinent, looking for clues and following them up before coming to a conclusion. He may order some tests to eliminate potential causes and establish positive results. He may also ask your continence adviser or district nurse to make a professional assessment of your incontinence. He will then be able to make a management plan, to see if continence can be wholly restored or greatly improved.

For example, the tests will tell him if you have diabetes or an infection – the most common cause of incontinence – or if you need to change any medicine you are taking. For an infection he will probably prescribe pills; for diabetes he will send you to a diabetic specialist, whilst keeping in touch with your progress.

After the menopause some women suffer from oestrogen deficiency, which can affect continence, so the doctor may consider oestrogen replacement therapy or the application of oestrogen cream.

The doctor will also find out if you suffer from stress incontinence and, if so, will send you to a gynaecologist and perhaps also to a physiotherapist. If he feels that your problems stem from prostate trouble, he may prescribe drugs and send you to a urological surgeon.

If the underlying cause is a problem common to the elderly, a geriatrician can help, in conjunction with a specialist physician or orthopaedic surgeon in the case of diseases such as arthritis or Parkinson's. In other cases somebody trained in the psychological side of medicine may be consulted.

Your continence adviser or district nurse, after making an assessment, will confer with your doctor, and will also give you immediate help and advice on all aspects of your problem.

A combination of any or all of these people may be called in to help restore continence.

Pelvic floor exercises are very valuable, and electrical treatment is used to re-educate both feeling and muscle-function.

The doctor will also be able to prescribe pads or appliances, either free or free from VAT; in many districts there is a National Health sheet washing service. He may, in addition, recommend that you start on a bladder retraining scheme or on exercise classes. If after treatment you are still finding difficulty in getting to the toilet, he may organise a home visit by an occupational therapist or a health visitor, to see if bars, handholds or ramps might help you in your home.

Depending on your circumstances, he may arrange for you to go to a day-centre; here you would get help and advice on all your problems, and it could relieve you of some of the strain. In some districts there is also a home-help service available.

There will no doubt be other ways in which your doctor can help.

DRUG THERAPY

Various drugs are prescribed to help recapture and maintain continence. They are taken in conjunction with the appropriate physical treatment described in this book: bladder retraining, pelvic floor exercises, use of vaginal cones, Functional Electrical Stimulation or Interferential Treatment and, of course, in support of surgery as needed.

Perhaps their most effective use at present is in treating people with unstable bladders, which contract too often and too easily, causing sudden total emptying, extreme urgency, frequency and bed wetting; the drugs are used to limit these contractions to normal levels.

Oxybutynin hydrochloride is effective as an antispasmodic, also calming nerve endings and acting as an analgesic and local anaesthetic; it has been used internationally for 15 years with success. A dry mouth may prove a side effect, but this can be avoided by starting the course with a very low dosage.

Propantheline helps to combat waste products in the bladder wall, but it is needed in quite high doses and so must be used with caution.

Different treatment is needed for stress incontinence, caused by weakness in the pelvic floor and the muscles at the neck of the bladder. The requirement here is a drug to make these muscles more effective.

Oestrogen therapy, taken orally, by patch or by implant can be effective for women after the menopause.

Phenylpropanolamine may be helpful, but it is available only in a mixture not obtainable on the National Health Service.

Oxybutynin hydrochloride is often helpful when stress incontinence includes an element of bladder instability, a not un-common occurrence.

Constant dribble incontinence is caused by the bladder's failing to contract, resulting in a permanently full bladder which overflows. This condition requires a drug to produce muscle contraction, a problem not easily solved.

Bethanechol chloride is used for this, but is not always effective.

An alternative approach is to reduce the resistance at the outlet of the bladder; **Prazosin** has been quite effective here.

HOW YOUR CONTINENCE ADVISER CAN HELP – GENERAL

In most areas there are continence advisers within the National Health Service. These are specialists who are there to help *all* incontinent people – and those looking after them – with any aspect of treatment and care. They work in close contact with doctors, with district nurses and with health, social and financial services. They hold clinics and conduct bladder training and retraining classes regularly in their areas, as well as organising education and assistance for sufferers, helpers and the general public.

In conjunction with the district nurses, who will look after you day by day if needed, continence advisers can make sure that you are getting the very best that the National Health Service offers, including the right appliances, garments and bedding. They can also monitor your condition and ensure that you are following the régime that suits you best. Whether you are a patient or a carer, do keep in regular touch with these specialists, who are highly skilled and also very approachable; do be completely frank, as they can help only if they know the true extent of your problems.

Your local continence adviser is there to help you personally and to ensure that your particular needs are provided for. The name and address of your nearest continence adviser can be obtained from the Association for Continence Advice, or send s.a.e. to

The Mead House, Sherborne, Glos. GL54 3DR.

CATHETERS

A catheter is a flexible, hollow tube with two holes near one end; this end is inserted into the bladder through the urethra, so that urine can drain down the tube into a bag or other container.

People who suffer from chronic incontinence, from whatever cause, may be advised by their doctor to use a catheter as a long-term measure. It will have a small bubble about an inch from the upper end, which is inflated with sterile water once it is in place; this stops it from slipping out of the bladder.

The catheter is then connected to a collection-bag strapped to the leg by soft, flexible straps or hung from the waist in a holster. The bag must always be lower than the bottom end of the catheter, to allow free drainage, and care must be taken that there are no kinks in the system. At night a stand or hanger is used by the bed, as the bag should not lie on the floor.

Bags are emptied through a tap at the bottom and flushed out with water before disposal. As with the insertion of any object foreign to the body, there is a risk of infection, so great care must be taken over personal washing. At first you may get occasional bladder cramps, but these should become less frequent. If there is leakage round the catheter, get in touch with your doctor during working hours. However, if no urine comes out, if you are in pain or if the urine appears abnormal, call your doctor at once.

There is now a catheter valve available which enables a sufferer to release urine when and where convenient, thus doing away with the necessity for bags.These are not suitable for everyone, so assessment by professionals is necessary.

Catheters are used also, as a short-term measure, after surgery or some accidents. Another, increasing, use of catheters is for intermittent self-catheterisation: when incontinence is caused by diminished communication between brain and bladder, or when the bladder is constantly full, your doctor or continence adviser may suggest this technique.

A plain catheter, without a bulb, is used, and the patient is taught the simple method of inserting it; the urine can be drained into a container or into the lavatory. The catheter is then withdrawn, washed and dried thoroughly and stored either in clean paper or in a bag supplied by the manufacturer. A catheter used this way will last from five days to a week.

The process is repeated every two to four hours; individuals will find their own best timing. Between catheterisations no pads are needed, and a much better quality of life is enjoyed. Thorough washing of hands, private parts and the catheter is essential, but can be kept simple; it is a clean, not a sterile, procedure.

GENERAL AND ELECTRICAL TREATMENT

Physiotherapists are very good at deciding on the right exercises in the right amounts for their patients. By regularly measuring the strength and performance of your muscles they can accurately assess improvement and then adjust the type, repetition and progression of exercises according to your personal need.

Another form of treatment is by electrical stimulation, which helps to re-educate both the 'feel' and the performance of the pelvic floor muscles. Extensive research and testing of this type of treatment is going on at present. The most usual type of stimulation is called Interferential Therapy, which makes muscles contract and relax. This treatment is given in an outpatient department, repeated regularly over a period of time.

An alternative treatment is called Functional Electrical Stimulation. The equipment for it is contained in a small portable box and, when the physiotherapist has shown you how it is operated, you can take it home and use it regularly for quite long periods. This treatment has proved very successful, but not many physiotherapy departments have enough equipment yet to lend out to all patients who need it.

There are two types of machine, one using a vaginal electrode, the other using external electrodes. Opinions about these vary widely among physiotherapists. External electrodes are more acceptable to many people, and the machines can be hired or bought more cheaply. Nevertheless, many experts believe that internal electrodes are greatly preferable.

Only a physiotherapist can say whether this would be a suitable treatment for you, and it does mean using the machine regularly for several hours – the more the better – for four to six months.

However, the machine can be used while carrying on normal everyday living, gradually restoring blood supply, nerves and muscles to proper function, so that the pelvic floor resumes its full tone and supportive function without tiring, and quick reaction for bladder-neck closure returns.

A great deal of the pelvic floor muscles' work is one of support; for this the muscular tone or tension must be good and the muscles must not tire easily. This means that the way you do your pelvic floor exercises is very important and should be based on the assessment scheme on page 35.

However, as well as their support function, the pelvic floor muscles have to contract, fast and immediately, to close the bladder neck for actions such as laughing or coughing, running or lifting. This means that pelvic floor exercises should be of two types, slow to build strength, and fast to stop disaster.

For people with unstable bladders pelvic floor exercises help because every time the pelvic floor contracts the bladder wall relaxes, thus helping to prevent urgency and dribbles.

Doing pelvic floor exercises effectively is difficult without moral support; this is where the physiotherapist can help enormously by encouragement, by helping with assessment and by choosing and using the right mixture of treatments, including for some, group exercises.

VAGINAL CONES

These are made of plastic or metal, in the shape of a cone provided with a tail like a tampon. They come in sets of three or five, graded according to weight. You insert the lightest cone into the vagina, as though it were a tampon, and see how long you can hold it in position by tightening your pelvic floor.

When you can hold the cone for five minutes, you try the next heavier one, and so on. This not only enables you to assess your progress, but also provides a very useful exercising aid for strengthening the pelvic floor. Cones can be provided by a physiotherapist, or you can buy them (see addresses at the end of the book).

PELVIC FLOOR EXERCISES

The pelvic floor muscles are exactly that: the floor that holds your bladder (and your uterus, if you are a woman) and intestines in place. This means that any weakness here causes trouble. These muscles do not form a flat, rigid floor; they are more like a sling or hammock hung from front to back; when they are weak, they tend to sag more.

They also reinforce the control of urine, surrounding the urethra and pressing on it when contracted. When the pelvic floor muscles contract, the bladder wall relaxes automatically, helping those with an unstable bladder to hold more urine. So do keep up these exercises, along with a retraining scheme.

Although in men the pelvic floor muscles surround only a short length of the urethra, it is enough to make a great difference to their continence, so these exercises are useful for men as well as for women.

It cannot be stressed too strongly that the exercises should be done very often for at least six months, but preferably for life.

The improvement will be gradual. At first it can be difficult to get the right 'feel'; many people believe that they are working their pelvic floor when, in fact, nothing at all is happening. It is therefore very important to assess this muscle activity properly. You can either do it yourself or get your physiotherapist or continence adviser to do it for you. It should be done at regular intervals, so that progress can be recorded and muscle strength measured.

EXERCISE 1

When you start this exercise, do it sitting on a hard chair, so that you can feel yourself against the seat.

1. Sit with your legs apart and lean forward with your elbows on your knees and your head drooped.

2. Consciously relax your stomach and buttock muscles.

3. Keeping these muscles relaxed, pull up the muscles round your back passage, as if trying to control diarrhoea, and hold on while you count slowly up to four. Then let go; try to let go even more and then tighten again as hard as you can. Hold and relax until you get a feeling of confidence about the exercise.

4. Next, thinking of the front passage, pull up the muscles as hard as you can, taking care not to tighten your stomach or buttock muscles. You will find this more difficult than with the back passage. Hold the muscle up as hard as you can while you count to four; then very consciously relax it. Think very hard about the relaxation, and see if you can let go even more; this contrast of tightening and relaxing makes it easier to get the right feeling for the exercise. Repeat this until you have a definite feeling of success, even if it is a small one to start with.

5. When you are sure of both areas, tighten both at the same time as hard as you can, hold for a count of four and relax. Repeat this about five times.

33

6. When you have managed this, try to pull up hard on the middle area, to get a lift from front to back; again, hold and relax about five times.

7. Now that you have mastered the different parts of the exercise, pull up on all three areas together and hold for a count of four, trying to get a feeling of real lift as well as tightening.

8. You can now simply do all three areas together. This can be done in any position anywhere, as long as you do it in accordance with your assessment and remember to do both a slow routine and a fast one.

9. **Most important**. Do your pelvic floor exercises with the same gaps for relaxation and time for recovery as in the assessment scheme, basing the number of contractions, length of hold and repeats on your findings. **Always** do slow contractions first.

10. Do these regularly, for example while driving to work or in the bath, but don't set yourself a ridiculous target. If you think three times a day is your maximum, be realistic. However, the more you do them the better, as long as there is a really good gap – at least an hour and a half – between bouts.

11. Assess yourself regularly and increase your exercise according to your findings. Thus, as your strength and reaction time increase, so do your exercises.

12. If you get little or no feeling of the exercises, go to your physiotherapist, who can help you with Functional Electrical Stimulation, cones or Interferential Therapy, as well as helping you with your routine.

EXERCISE 2

If you ever have any feeling of hesitancy about beginning a stream, do not do this exercise. Some experts do not now include it, but for most people, if used only once a day, it is helpful.

As you urinate, try to stop the stream. Don't try this first thing in the morning and, to begin with, try it towards the end of the stream. Gradually work this up until you are starting and stopping three to four times, and near the beginning of the stream as well, but only on one toilet visit daily.

1. Read carefully the section headed 'Exercise 1' on the previous page and practise it until you think you have the 'feel'.

2. Insert two fingers into the vagina, either forward and back or from side to side, and spread them until there is a snug fit.

3. Lift your pelvic floor and feel the contraction on your fingers; now give yourself a grade from 0 to 5 for the amount of movement; 0 = no movement, 1 = a flicker, 2 = very weak, 3 = weak, 4 = fair, 5 = strong.

4. After a rest do this again and see for how long a count you can hold the contraction, from 0-10 seconds.

5. After an interval do the same again and see how many times you can repeat the squeeze and hold, before your muscle will not hold any more, allowing a gap of 5-10 seconds between contractions.

   You will now have assessed yourself, for example:

   (a) at grade 2 for strength,

   (b) at a count of 5 seconds for contraction,

   (c) able to repeat the exercise 6 times. This is recorded as 2/5/6.

6. Now go through the assessment programme with fast contractions, giving yourself grades for flickers, quickness of reaction, hold and repeat times. This is important.

   You now have two assessments, one for slow exercises and one for fast.

Then, each time you do your pelvic floor exercises, you should base them on these findings, trying to achieve 5 seconds 6 times at intervals of at least 1½ hours. Assess yourself and, if you can improve on any of the figures, try for the better figure next time, for example 6 seconds 7 times, and also record when you have managed a grade 3 strength.

When you think that you have improved markedly in any part of either fast or slow exercises, assess yourself again; then try for a higher figure next time.

Any now, also very important –

35

HOW YOU CAN HELP YOURSELF

The main aim of this book is to help you to be independent in your own home, so that you do not have to rely on residential care.

However, if you are in a residential home, some of the practical tips and exercises may still be valuable.

In either case, you may need support from your family and friends and from professional people. Your family and friends may find some points in this book which will help them to help you.

MIND OVER MATTER

1. If you want to reduce incontinence by helping yourself, *you must want to do so strongly enough.* This may mean that you have to rethink your priorities and be prepared to apply the determination and effort required. But, whatever you decide, many ways of easing your problems are explained in this book, besides the demanding but valuable retraining schemes and exercises.

2. Following a bladder retraining scheme and doing the exercises will require self-control and perseverance, as well as altering some of your habits.

3. Your positive attitude to becoming more aware of your own body and to reducing your incontinence will be a key factor in achieving success.

4. Many people have to adjust to the idea of having a goal to aim at; all the retraining schemes are progressive, and you will find that aiming at realistic goals becomes part of your life for three or four months.

5. For people with extreme urgency this may well be a time of discomfort; you may need new diversions to engage your attention.

6. Anxiety, stress and fear may be contributory causes of frequency, so any way of reducing tensions will be helpful.

7. Get into the habit of thinking and planning ahead.

8. If you rely on other people to get you to a toilet, try to arrange with them when it will be convenient. If you can arrange things beforehand, and yet be a little flexible, it will help you not to

worry and allow the people looking after you to organise their time. On the other hand, if a helper is near and not too busy, it may be a good idea to seize the opportunity, rather than trying to hang on.

9. If your day seems a bit monotonous, try to divide it up with a highlight, however small, in each part.

10. Watch your weight. Being overweight can be demoralising, and it also puts an extra strain on the pelvic floor muscles. If this is a problem, get help with your diet; ask your doctor for the right diet sheets and, if you need help with the discipline of keeping to it, try either attending classes or finding a friend who also needs to diet, to compare notes.

11. The strength and tone of all the body muscles are important for your health and well-being. Even if you cannot go out, try to follow the course of exercises on pages 56 to 58. Stronger pelvic floor and stomach muscles will help the bladder to empty more efficiently.

12. People who are deaf or find it difficult to communicate should have a bell or other device to signal for what they need.

SHARING PROBLEMS

1. Share your anxieties, if you can, with a reliable person. It may be somebody outside the family, the continence adviser or the district nurse.

2. Find another incontinence sufferer, so that you can share your knowledge without embarrassment and find ways to help each other. You could compare notes on exercises, eating and drinking habits, protective clothing and so on. This will help to dispel the sense of isolation which people often feel.

SOME HINTS FOR HELPERS

1. A sympathetic understanding of problems will be appreciated, but matter-of-fact, practical help is more important.

2. Do practice the exercises *with* the patient; doing things together makes life much easier.

3. You may be the right person to remind the patient about exercises, toilet training and keeping charts of progress.

4. Even if the person you are helping is beyond pelvic floor or retraining exercises, charting the urinary patterns will help you to time toilet visits or bed-panning, thus reducing discomfort and enabling you to plan your time. Also, success in remaining dry may increase the patient's self-respect. Anything you can do to stimulate mental processes will make the patient happier and your job more valuable and interesting.

5. Try to find another sufferer who can share experience and compare progress with the patient.

6. If you are the regular helper, it is much better to mention a wet patch or a problem with smell, rather than leave the patient to find out later and be embarrassed in company.

7. Patients are often anxious about getting to the toilet in time, so try to think ahead.

8. Always have enough supplies of pads and garments ready for an emergency and arrange their washing and disposal in the easiest way for both of you.

9. Most people prefer to be independent, but some may need positive encouragement to do as much as possible for themselves. Finding a way to persuade them without seeming "bossy" will demand quite a lot of imagination.

10. Independent-minded people may be reluctant to ask for help, and here too imagination and a knowledge of the patient will enable you to do the right thing at the right time without being asked.

11. Stimulation of a purely social kind, such as going out and meeting people, can make a *real* difference to a patient's determination to manage difficulties better.

12. Nearly all patients are sensitive about "being a trouble", and so react strongly to any hint of superiority or being patronised. A cheerful and whole-hearted approach works wonders.

13. Make your help as unobtrusive as possible; having to feel grateful all the time is a great burden.

14. All of us at some time will feel our patience sorely tried, nerves getting frayed, irritation even resulting in loss of temper. Don't bottle it up, as that can make the situation worse. However awkward it may seem, talk about it with the patient.

15. Take time off, and be a little protectively selfish. The relief that comes from doing your own thing, even for a short while, is well worth organising, and it will benefit not only yourself but your patient. Take a look at the BBC booklet *Who Cares?*, which has many ideas and the names of societies which provide cover (also given at the back of this book).

16. Try to find other helpers with whom you can pool ideas; they may have thought of ways of helping which haven't occurred to you, and vice versa.

17. Listen to all the advice you can, but avoid being over-persuaded into methods of care which don't come naturally to you; there are many ways of helping and, in the end, you will probably be most effective in your own particular style.

18. If you can't achieve perfection, neither can anyone else, but these points are worth bearing in mind.

19. Finally, do use the help available from the National Health Service, remembering that the district nurse and continence adviser are there to help you.

FINANCIAL PROBLEMS

1. Do get all the assistance that you are entitled to. It may seem confusing and difficult to discover what help is available, financial or otherwise but, if you are not satisfied, *don't give up*; your local continence adviser, district nurse or doctor will point you in the right direction. There is a list of agencies and books on pages 80 to 84.

2. There may be charitable trusts, either local or national, which can provide help with washing machines, dryers and laundry expenses. Try the agencies listed at the end of this book.

3. If you work or are connected with a large organisation, or have retired from one, write to the head of the relevant personnel division; there is almost always support available from big firms, such as ICI, and organisations, such as the Church, the Civil Service, armed forces, trade unions and so on.

4. If you cannot manage to go to the toilet, dress or cook for yourself, or if you need constant attention, you may be entitled to a Constant Attendance Allowance. You or your helpers or the social

worker can get in touch with the Department of Health or of Social Security, which will send an independent doctor to assess your needs. There are two levels of allowance, one for daytime care and another for 24-hour care, both tax-free. Keep a record of toilet visits and your night-time attendance over a period, and don't understate your problems. If your helper is of working age and you are receiving a Constant Attendance Allowance, then your helper may be eligible for an Invalid Care Allowance. Remember that, if you are receiving any additional benefits, the amount of the Care Allowance will be deducted from them; on the other hand, it does give your helper very good pension rights, so it is worth considering carefully. If you are on Income Support (IS), you may get an income support grant or loan from the social fund to pay for bedding, washing machine etc. Your local DSS will give you Form SF.300.

NB. *Much of the above paragraph may change in April 1993. A six-monthly* update can be obtained from The Mead House, Sherborne, Glos. GL54 3DR or from DIG (see end of book).

SENSIBLE TOILET RULES – DAYTIME

1. Go to the toilet at sensible intervals; if you feel the need to go very often, try to lengthen the intervals gradually. On the other hand, if you find that you have accidents because for years you have been used to going for long periods without visiting the toilet, discipline yourself to go more frequently, *go before you really want to.*

2. Try to get your bladder as empty as possible every time you go. Here are one or two suggestions:

    (a) When you feel you have finished, put your clenched hand against your lower stomach and tighten the muscles hard; then bend over and try to push out more urine.

    (b) Try coughing when bent over; this will often bring more urine down.

    (c) For women – press a tissue firmly against yourself and wait a few seconds; often more urine will come.

    (d) For men – press the base of the penis below the scrotum and milk down the whole length of the penis.

(e) For men especially – but also for women – wait for a minute or two, and this may have the same result.

(f) Try moving about then starting again.

3. A rest with your feet raised will increase urine production, so a rest after lunch may help to keep you dry later.

4. Make sure you have the way to the toilet clear of chairs, small rugs and other obstructions.

5. In the toilet, ensure that the layout is as helpful as possible. The seat should be at the right height; supports should be available for getting up, and there should be no slippery rugs or hard angles.

6. Wear clothes which are as simple as possible, not only for comfort but for ease in taking them off. Make sure also that clothing is not too tight around the waist or over the lower stomach, as this will cause pressure on the bladder.

7. Pre-menstrual days are usually worse for stress incontinence, so take this into account.

8. Make a note of (a) what period of time after a drink, and (b) how large a drink, makes a visit to the toilet necessary. Then try to space out your drinks at times convenient for that particular day. Use your Chart 1 to verify the times and quantities and, if you know you are going out in the afternoon, alter your drinks pattern accordingly. Remember that it may take several days of careful charting before you find a pattern.

9. If you take medicines, such as water pills, note on your chart how this affects your toilet pattern and time your pills to fit in with your day's programme.

SENSIBLE TOILET RULES – NIGHT TIME

1. Go to the toilet before you go upstairs, then again just before getting into bed, making sure your bladder is as empty as possible.

2. A walk last thing at night, for those who can take one, sometimes helps, even if it is only round the house.

3. Notice if a late drink makes a difference and, if so, alter your habit. Use your Chart 1 to help you experiment to find the best drinking habits for you, and record times of urinating at night. Perhaps when you wake up in the night might be a better time for a sip or two from your thermos.

4. A commode by your bed may be a help, or a chamber-pot well fixed on a low chair. For men, a urine bottle, as used in hospitals, may be the answer.

5. If you take medicines, such as water pills, note on your chart how this affects your toilet patterns and time your pills to work just before bedtime.

6. It is entirely normal for an elderly person to have to go to the toilet during the night, so make it as easy for yourself as you can.

7. If you can manage to alter your habit and empty your bowels before going to bed rather than in the morning, this will reduce pressure on the bladder.

8. If wetting your bed wakes you up, look at the time and try setting your alarm for half or three-quarters of an hour before this. If this is not successful, try an hour or an hour and a half earlier.

9. Have spare pads and padded squares handy, so that you can make yourself comfortable, and remember to have a container, with a lid, for disposal of used pads within easy reach of your bed or commode.

10. Try wearing top-half-only nightwear, or a short nightie or one that opens down the back, so that you can change a pad and be comfortable without changing night clothes.

11. If you often find yourself wet when you wake up, read pages 44 and 45, which has advice about drinks and medicines, and pages 45 and 46 about sleeping patterns. Do tell your doctor.

GOING OUT

1. Always go to the toilet before you go out.

2. Be on the safe side; if your incontinence is not very bad but can embarrass you, wear a stick-on superabsorbent pad.

3. Carry with you a spare pair of pants with pads, a packet of wet wipes and a plastic bag.

4. Other alternatives, and I think good ones, are the reusable pants with a built-in one-way-wet pad. These can be washed as normal pants and last about a year, suitable for light to medium incontinence. They are made to look like normal briefs or bikinis, the men's like normal Y-fronts – invaluable for men with dribbles.

Makers' names and addresses are at the end of the book.

5.   A bottle or a woman's collapsible appliance, which fits the contours of the body and is *unspillable* and disposable, kept in the car, can save the day on a journey. See page 86 for stockist or maker.

6.   When you are in other people's houses, make sure you ask where the toilet is, so that there is the least possible delay if you need it.

7.   Another cause for anxiety is the possibility of wetting a chair when away from home. Many people with bad backs take a cushion with them and you might consider doing the same yourself. A square pad enclosed in an attractive, washable cotton cover need not draw attention and will make you feel secure, whether with family or friends or in a car or restaurant.

8.   If you are away from home and are drinking alcohol, remember that this will tend to lessen your control, so make sure that you go to the toilet during your visit and just before you leave.

9.   Get to know your area and find out where there are public toilets, shops, hotels or pubs that can be used. Try to plan your shopping so that one of these can be reached easily if necessary.

10.   When you pass a toilet, consider whether it would be sensible to use it, even if you don't need to, as the next may be too far away.

11.   Bus steps are high, and raising your leg to that height may need care in order to avoid a leak.

12.   If you suffer from stress incontinence, avoid stepping sideways when shopping. Turn sideways on to the shelf and move forward that way. Tighten your pelvic muscles, or at least exert control before moving.

13.   Be careful about bending over, as this causes extra pressure on the bladder. The same is true about lifting things.

14.   If you are in a car, bumpy roads and vibration may affect your bladder, so pad up in case.

15.   If you are going out next day, be a little flexible about your routines and plan them to make things as secure as possible, using your Chart 1.

16.   If you have a catheter or penile appliance, do see that you start off with an empty bag and also that your holster for the bag is comfortable and in the most convenient place.

1.   If you are about to get up after sitting for some time, tighten your pelvic muscles before moving, and then get up slowly.

2.   When you have got to your feet, move gradually and don't hurry.

3.   If you feel that you are about to sneeze or cough, stand still, cross your legs, pull up your pelvic floor muscles, tighten your buttocks, and you are then in the best position to resist loss of control.

4.   If a cough is coming while you are sitting down – either indoors or in a car – lean back, stretch your legs and then pull up the pelvic floor.

5.   It is important to go to the toilet not only before sexual intercourse, but afterwards, as this helps to avoid cystitis.

6.   Any movement which means moving your legs further apart, either forwards or sideways, makes leaks more likely.

7.   Lifting and bending also can cause leaks.

8.   If you know that, for you, certain movements are bound to cause leaks, think ahead and try to avoid them as much as possible, or prepare yourself by tightening your pelvic floor muscles before doing them.

9.   If you are suddenly overcome with extreme urgency when moving, stand still for a minute and lift your pelvic floor; think positively about control, and then move slowly, with small steps, to the toilet.

10.   When you get to the toilet, try very hard not to rush; pull down pants and position yourself with as little movement as possible.

11.   Remember that it is at the very door of the house, or in similar situations of imminent relief, that accidents most often happen, because you feel safe and so relax.

TIMING OF DRINKS AND MEDICINES

1.   **Drink enough.** Many people think that restricting their fluid intake will help their problem, but **the opposite is true.** Restricted drinking causes:

(a) Constipation. This is a major contributory cause of incontinence, and drinking is a natural laxative, much better than pills and other remedies.

(b) Over-concentrated urine. Any drugs you may be taking, caffeine or harmful materials in the urine will naturally have more effect and can increase urgency by irritation.

You should drink 8-12 cups of fluid a day.

2. Use your Chart 1 to help you time your drinking, especially later in the day, if you have trouble at night.

3. Note if the amounts taken at any one time are significant, and experiment by using the chart.

4. Again, use Chart 1 to see if the timing of medicines is significant.

5. For some people, no pattern will emerge, in which case try to be as regular as possible with your drinking habits.

6. Fizzy drinks, tea, coffee or anything containing caffeine irritate the bladder, so don't drink too much of them. This does *not* mean don't drink them at all, but decaffeinated coffee and weaker tea may be helpful. In extreme cases your doctor will advise.

7. Alcohol not only relaxes muscle but it reduces your awareness and slows down reaction, so remember that you will be more incontinent than usual after drinking it.

8. Some drugs, such as pain-killers and muscle-relaxants, reduce muscular tone and so increase incontinence. Your doctor might change your medicines if he knew you were taking them.

9. There are drugs that can help some types of incontinence, so do talk to your doctor.

10. When you learn more from your Chart 1 about the time-lapses between drinks and toilet visits, discuss them with your helper, so that you can plan convenient times together.

11. Sleeping pills. Many people are incontinent at night because these pills cause them to sleep through urinating. There are pills which help you to sleep, but not so deeply or for a shorter time. Consult your doctor. *Do you really need sleeping pills?*

SUGGESTIONS ABOUT SLEEPING PATTERNS FOR THE ELDERLY

As people grow older, they sleep for shorter periods, so it is natural to have quite long spells when you are awake at night. Do you really need those sleeping pills? Why not make up your mind to reorganise yourself and sleep only when you really feel the need to? You will always get enough sleep.

For instance, if you fall asleep in your chair after supper, you may not want or need to sleep again until, say, 1 a.m. If you live alone or have a separate bedroom, there is no problem. You can take your knitting, a book, a radio with headphones, writing materials etc. and sit cosily in bed with something round your shoulders until you feel sleepy; then go to the toilet, return to bed and turn out the light.

Suppose you wake at 5 a.m.; if you live in a household with others, they will not be up yet, so go to the toilet again, have a small hot drink from a thermos by your bed and plan the day ahead.

You could do some of the exercises described in this booklet, think about your family or neighbours, sort out your problems, if you have any, as far as you can, read a little, turn on the radio or do some mending, and by 7.30 you might feel sleepy again. Go to the toilet, come back to bed and drop off until 8.30 or 9.00. It won't really matter if it is 10.30, *so long as you don't worry about it*. Then, when you want to sleep during the day, don't feel guilty; remember you have that amount of time free at night.

All this is, of course, not easy if you live in a residential or nursing home, but people are much more understanding nowadays; a radio with headphones or a small spotlight by your bed need not disturb others, even though mealtimes and waking and bed-times may be inflexible. The night-nurse will get to know your habits and, if you explain the problem, she will help you. She would much rather bring a bedpan or help you to the toilet than change a sopping bed or cope with the soreness that results from sitting in urine. Almost always, a routine emerges, and a nurse will soon know at what hour to come and look after you.

You may well find it difficult to change the habits of a lifetime; it will require a positive effort of mental adjustment and it may take a little time but, if this system enables you to do without sleeping pills, it will help you to be more continent.

HELP WITH SEXUAL PROBLEMS

Everybody wants to enjoy a normal sex-life, and anything that makes for awkwardness, embarrassment or inability may be an obstacle for both parties. An understanding of your incontinence will help you to explain your difficulty to your partner. In some cases, reading about problems and how they can be overcome proves helpful.

I recommend a book called *Entitled to Love* by Dr Wendy Greengrass, which is available from SPOD, the Association to aid Sexual and Personal Relationships for people with a Disability. The address is at the end of this book, and SPOD will help with other suggestions for reading and will give individual advice.

Any condition which impairs blood or nerve supply to the sexual organs – such as spinal injury or diabetes – may cause difficulty, impotence or lack of orgasm. Weak or damaged pelvic floor muscles and a bladder which spasms, or retains urine, can cause leakage during intercourse. Bed wetting causes great anxieties, and some people have other physical handicaps to overcome, but perhaps the most elusive problem is the psychological feeling of being different; great sensitivity and understanding are needed here.

HERE ARE SOME HINTS WHICH MAY BE HELPFUL:

If you have been incontinent, wash yourself or have a bath.

Make yourself as comfortable as possible, with support which will make the most of your mutual abilities.

Try to use positions where pressure is not put on the bladder.

Empty your bowels and bladder as completely as possible before intercourse.

Remove catheters, if you can; if not, make them secure up the penis or on the thigh. A heavy duty condom can be worn over a catheter.

Drugs and implants to help to keep a penis erect are now available; consult your doctor.

Lubrication always helps.

Great satisfaction can be obtained without the penis's entering the vagina.

Do make every effort to strengthen your pelvic floor muscles; this will increase your continence and give greater satisfaction to both partners.

Don't hesitate to ask for professional advice if you need it.

Children with severe mental and physical handicaps, suffering from consequent chronic incontinence, need all the help they can possibly get, and so do their helpers. There may be one or two points in various other sections which could be valuable to them, but remember that these children suffer also from social and psychological problems, as other children do. The following section deals primarily with the less severely handicapped child, but some of these hints might help the severely handicapped as well.

Some children are much slower than others to become toilet-trained, and this can be a great anxiety for parents. It has become clear that children's urinary systems develop at varying rates, and the rate seems to run in families. Boys tend to develop later than girls; many children are not reliably continent, because of their structural capacity, until the age of 11 to 13. It may be hard to discover the reason without making the child too self-conscious and aware of being different.

The cause may be medical, or it may be more social and psychological; examples of this are given below. In either case, don't hesitate to consult your doctor and/or local continence adviser. Opinions vary about the best course of action, so the suggestions you receive will depend on the views of your adviser. There is probably no single correct method so, if one way does not work, try another. But three things are clear:

(a)   you know the character of your child best, as well as the day-to-day pressures of family, of school and of growing up. This knowledge, applied with love and common sense, is vital in getting to the heart of the problem;

(b)   it is unwise and counter-productive to punish, humiliate or scold a child unduly;

(c)   it is often helpful to suggest achievement goals, with encouragement and praise when possible.

FACTS WORTH NOTING:

1.   More boys than girls have toilet problems.

2.   The older the child is before the problem is acknowledged, the harder it is to cure.

3.   For children who are incontinent throughout the 24 hours, once the daytime problem is solved the night-time problem usually improves dramatically.

4.   Laziness and habit are very often contributory causes.

5.   A need to draw attention to themselves, commonly subconscious, often causes children to wet or dirty their pants.

6.   Hidden fears can be a cause, and anxieties, such as a new baby, a change of school or divorce in the family can make a dry child revert.

7.   Some fact, apparently entirely unrelated, such as dislike or fear of a person, or a longing to possess something of their own, may cause children to remain incontinent.

8.   Anxiety about wetting a bed can cause a child to keep awake and so lead to a pattern of sleeplessness.

9.   Some other physical disorder, such as diabetes, can aggravate an existing problem.

10.   A feeling of inferiority, however unjustified or unnecessary, can be the source of the trouble.

11.   Bed-wetting can remain a problem into adulthood, but many of the sufferers are high achievers.

12.   Teenage sufferers frequently hide and hoard underpants and sheets.

13.   Fear of embarrassment and loss of face among friends of their own age can cause a sense of isolation, and may adversely affect their school work and their behaviour.

14.   For teenagers bed-wetting can become a fixation, causing an intense anxiety which makes the problem worse.

15.   The positive and supportive attitude of parents, especially if the problem continues into the late teens, will make a big contribution towards a cure.

SOME HINTS ABOUT BED-WETTING

Decide with your adviser whether to adopt the unobtrusive or the positive action approach.

UNOBTRUSIVE ACTION

6.   Don't use talcum powder or deodorants between the legs; both can be irritant.

7.   You may be allergic to scented soaps; if so, use one of the plain soaps now available.

8.   If you start to get sore and are not wearing pads, try changing your washing powder to *Lux* and rinsing garments extra well.

9.   If soreness continues, don't buy fancy creams or ointments, but ask your doctor for something. Zinc and castor oil cream is as good as anything, short of a doctor's prescription.

10.   If you have cortisone cream or ointment, which may have been prescribed for you, *never* use it on a broken skin.

11.   If you have been fitted with a catheter or penile appliance, your district nurse will instruct you, but the general guidelines for hygiene apply. Look out especially for soreness and don't ignore it.

MANAGEMENT OF SMELL

1.   Smell is one of the main causes of embarrassment to incontinent people; there is no substitute for keeping as clean as possible.

2.   Take care about your clothes, which are very important. They should be simple to manage and not too tight, easily washed and dried. Try wearing "top-only" night clothes and change all clothes as often as possible.

3.   Materials of man-made fibres are the easiest to wash but, after a time, however well they are washed, they retain smell in a way that natural fibres, such as cotton, do not. When weighing up the advantages, it is as well to be aware of this.

4.   Remember to wash whenever you have become wet.

5.   Do change your pads often enough; it is when air gets to urine that it really begins to smell.

6.   Make sure that at home your bed is covered with a waterproof material which does not move or become crumpled; fitted covers for all standard-sized mattresses are available from *Boots* and other big chemists. See also addresses at the back of the book. Remember to wash this cover with disinfectant, as it will retain smell if stale urine is left on the surface.

7.   When there is severe incontinence at night, top bedclothes can get

wet even with the best of pads and garments, so do use washable duvets or sheets and blankets that can be washed easily.

8.   A plastic or vinyl sheet under a washable rug at your bedside is a good idea, as it is often when you move after sleep that a leak occurs. These too will need washing as necessary. **Do ensure that the rug is anchored in some way, so that it cannot slip.**

9.   Put the chair and chamber-pot by your bed, on a big enough washable surface. The chair should be washable too, and it must be safe from tipping or sliding; a commode is ideal. Do have a lid for your chamber-pot.

10.   Don't be tempted to have a carpet in the toilet. Accidental spills happen very easily and can't be fully wiped from a carpet, so the smell increases.

11.   Air your rooms very well, not forgetting the toilet.

12.   If you are wearing waterproof or one-way-wet pants, they must be washed as often as they are wet.

13.   For men with dribbling problems, remember that urine acts as a bleaching agent, and discoloration of clothing happens quickly. After finishing the stream, remember to wait until there is another small flow, and this should avoid wetting the trousers. Then follow the procedure on page 22. If you do wet your trousers, the sooner they are washed, the less likely they are to be stained. If it happens regularly, it is sensible to wear trousers of a washable material, such as corduroy.

14.   Upholstery retains smell and is not easy to clean, so it may be best for your favourite easy chair to be covered in vinyl, with a cotton pad on top for comfort. Another method is to have a plastic sheet big enough to tuck in well all round and come a little way up the back and sides of the chair; this can be kept in place by a larger throw-over cotton cloth which will overhang the back and arms. It goes without saying that the plastic, whether cover or sheet, will need regular wiping down or washing, as will the cotton pad or cover. For washable chair pads, see end of book.

15.   As with getting out of bed, getting up from a chair may cause accidents. If you know that this happens, it is sensible to have a washable rug or an easily wiped surface under your chair.

16.   Do wash your chamber-pot or bottle well enough, using some disinfectant.

Deciding that pads are necessary is a big step to take, and many women put off this decision for far too long, in spite of suffering anxiety about the appearance of wet patches in public.

Men also tend to ignore wet patches from dribbling, and it is surprising how often they will continue to wear discoloured trousers, pretending that nothing is wrong; even their wives seem unwilling to point out the problem.

When incontinence is more severe, and urgency makes accidents frequent, something has to be done. A wide range of protective garments are available in the following combinations:

(a)   reusable pants and pads,
(b)   reusable pants with disposable pads,
(c)   disposable pants and pads.

Bedding and furniture protectors, such as chair or cushion covers, can also be reusable or disposable.

You will find out by trial and error what suits you and your helpers best, but *do* get advice from your continence adviser or district nurse. The National Health Service provides a wide variety of pants, pads and bedding, but it is also a good idea to know what is available and to have an adaptable selection ready for all occasions; for example, if you go away for two days, you may have to use disposables all the time.

Your washing facilities and your ability to cope with heavy garments will influence your choice, as will the cost. Remember that there are organisations which can help with washing machines, clothes dryers and electricity bills (see Agencies on pages 80 and 81). As well as the ordinary tumble dryers and outdoor clothes-lines, cabinet dryers, racks that fit over heaters or radiators and ceiling racks on pulleys are worth considering.

There is a list of articles in general use, showing the circumstances in which they are useful, starting on page 84. There is also an explanation of an absorbent bed-sheet, which is used without padded garments.

MANAGEMENT AND DISPOSAL OF PADS AND GARMENTS

You may well have your own arrangements already, but some people have found these suggestions helpful.

AT HOME

Two containers with lids are needed, one lined with a plastic binliner, the other provided with a bucket. Pedal bins are very useful for this, although any waterproof container with a lid will do.

When you are changing underclothes, if the pad is *very* wet, wrap it in a newspaper before placing it in the bin with the plastic liner. When the liner is full, tie the neck and put it into a heavy-duty dustbin liner. This can be kept in a dustbin and will be collected in the normal way. Never try to flush even small pads down the toilet.

Soiled ordinary pants or pad-holding pants can be put in the second bin and then soaked in water, if possible with *Napisan* or the equivalent; this reduces smell, and the pants will then need only rinsing according to the instructions on the packet. Night clothes and reusable pads can be treated in the same way, but this method may not be suitable for outer garments, as dyes can run and manmade fibres deteriorate in this kind of solution.

Some areas have a disposal service: ring your social services department.

Vernon Carus supply a good unit that contains and keeps soiled pads (see end of book).

AWAY FROM HOME

Bins for pads are provided in public toilets, and pants can be put in a polythene bag in your handbag. A newspaper also may come in handy, as well as spare pads and pants; all-in-one disposable garments have the advantage that you need not carry any soiled garment home.

If you are visiting a private house, it is better to have *two* plastic bags, because it is more satisfactory to separate the wet pad from the pants at once, though of course if you are using disposable all-in-one garments, only one bag is needed.

Wet wipes and a spare towel also may be useful.

Your general health and muscle tone are important, so do take regular exercise. Here are four simple rules for everyone to follow:

1. Start your exercise routine gently, so that you work without strain, within your capabilities.

2. Do persevere and keep going; it is a good idea to set aside a definite time for exercises.

3. Increase the length of time and the severity of the exercises over a period.

4. Recognise a sensible summit and avoid objectives beyond your reach; work up to a level of exercise which suits your lifestyle.

Suggestions for the Younger Person

(Especially for Women After Childbirth)

1. A series of exercises, as advocated for slimming and general wellbeing, often use muscles that help and complement the pelvic floor muscles. There are many published routines available.

2. Swimming is an excellent general exercise.

3. A selected number of women tried using a rowing-machine, and at the same time doing pelvic floor exercises. All were incontinent when they started, and after three months *every one* showed a marked improvement. The strength of the pelvic floor is a major factor in continence, and exercising the muscles used in rowing evidently gives useful support.

4. Do **avoid** heavy lifting or exercise that adds strain to the pelvic floor, as over-exercising weak muscles can damage them.

Suggestions for the Housebound or Elderly

Read through the list of exercises below and decide which are within your capabilities; your doctor or district nurse, a relative or friend might be a good person to discuss this with.

You don't have to do all the exercises; perhaps you can build up to them.

If you get breathless, don't overdo it; do less, consult your doctor.

If you find an exercise painful, don't persevere without referring to your doctor.

Do find someone to exercise with you if possible, especially to begin with.

1. Lie down on a firm surface and think about each part of your body in turn. Be methodical; start at your head or feet and work up or down, trying to be aware of every part of yourself. You can, of course, do this in any position, but the touch of the surface against you will help your awareness. If you lose your concentration, give it a rest and then try again, starting where you left off. In a few days you should be able to achieve awareness of your whole body.

2. Once again starting at either head or feet, tighten the muscles of one foot, or of your face, as hard as you can, hold for a count of two and then relax. Think very hard about the relaxation and see if, by thinking, you can let go even more. Keeping your eyes shut may help you to concentrate. Work through the parts of your body separately, one by one. If you feel daunted by the thought of your whole body, concentrate on the following.
    (a) the muscles at the back of your neck,
    (b) pulling your shoulder-blades together,
    (c) the muscles that arch your back in the middle,
    (d) your buttocks,
    (e) your stomach muscles
    (f) the muscles above your knees, which are used to straighten them,
    (g) your pelvic floor muscles.
         Do this just once to begin with, but increase the number of times to five or six and the length of time you hold to a count of four or five; each time try to get a greater contrast between tightening and relaxing. Many people find that concentrated effort to relax from just being aware of your muscles is a great help in getting to sleep.

3. Take two or three really deep breaths, from as deep in your chest as possible, and blow out every bit of air you can. *Don't* increase the number of these breaths taken at any one time, but try to take two or three at more frequent intervals during the day.

4. Unless you have been told not to, try once every day to move your joints through as full a range of movement as you can without pain. Do start gently, and stop if it feels painful, but gradually build up to two or three full movements and see if you can achieve a rather greater range of movement as time goes on. If you are in doubt about the wisdom of exercising any particular joint, consult your doctor or district nurse first.

5. *Gently* try to stretch your whole body, and then relax again. Breathe evenly as you do this, and stop if you find it painful.

You need not do all these exercises at once, but you might try short sessions with one area of your body periodically during the day.

BLADDER RETRAINING

It may come as a surprise to learn that incontinence can be overcome by retraining toilet habits; in fact, so many people have managed to improve the quality of their lives in this way that it is well worth making the effort.

It is only fair to warn you that it is often difficult, that you will have set-backs and that *you must want the result strongly enough to persevere*. If you accept the challenge and are equal to it, you will feel that your struggle has been well rewarded.

The retraining period will probably take between 10 and 16 weeks, but it varies considerably from one person to another.

If there are retraining classes in your area, do join them if you can; they may have different ways of retraining and different charts, but the principle will be the same. Naturally you should follow whatever method is being used by the class.

An Important Reminder

1. **Keep up your pelvic floor exercises. Every time your pelvic floor muscles are worked, your bladder automatically relaxes, making it easier for you to hold more urine and thus have less urgency.**

2. Drink enough – about 8 to 12 cups a day.

3. Avoid drinks that you know make your frequency greater.

4. Avoid irritant soap powders and "biological" washing powders.

5. When you are trying to extend the intervals between your toilet

visits, find some interesting activity to occupy your mind, such as reading, sewing, cooking, watching television, etc.

6.   Wear clothes which are loose and easy to manage.

7.   Expect to fail sometimes and don't get too depressed.

8.   Get some help or company if you can.

9.   Try sitting on a rolled-up towel or on your foot, as this will help support your pelvic floor and increase your awareness of your bladder.

10.   Empty your bowels regularly.

Keep a strict record for at least three days, noting the amounts as in Chart 1. For most people a clear pattern will emerge. For some people, if there is no regular time pattern, a pattern of high production of urine related to certain activities or circumstances may emerge. For a few there will be no pattern. Look carefully at your charts and put the pattern that becomes clear on the blank chart at the back of the book under "present pattern" – only amounts of urine are needed; see page 26 as an example of what should go on Chart 2.

What you do next depends on the pattern, or lack of it, that you have found.

GROUP A

Those people who have to make frequent and urgent visits to the toilet, with a time pattern.

You have a bladder that is very sensitive to the presence of urine, and it contracts to expel this urine far too often. You have to learn to suppress these contractions, enabling you to hold more urine for longer periods. In order to help you lengthen these periods, you will need Chart 2, marked in quarter-hours and shown on page 90. In the left-hand column put your present pattern of production of urine taken from Chart 1.

Group A1. If you can't hold on for as long as an hour, make marks every hour on your chart, and go at the hour whether you want to or not, *but not in between.*

Group A2. If on average you can hold on for an hour or more, increase this time by a quarter of an hour and enter in the second column the new pattern which you are aiming to achieve. Go to the toilet at these times whether you want to or not, *but not in between.*

Then each day for a week, fill in the next column, and this will show you what progress you are making.

Note your night patterns, if possible.

Now note the following points:

(a) Follow your new routine until you are able to do so *easily* and remain dry without undue strain. Complete one week in any case, recording success or failure and also times when you find it difficult to hold on and times when it is easier.

(b) Still keeping your record, repeat this for another week, or until you are successful. If at certain times of day you regularly find it impossible to hold on,

    (i) look back to your drink chart (Chart 1) see if it relates to this difficulty; if so, try altering the time or amount of the drink;

    (ii) shorten your time allowance by a quarter of an hour, *at this time of day only.*

If at other times it is really easy to succeed, add a quarter of an hour to the time interval. These procedures allow a natural pattern to evolve.

(c) *If* you find that you are not succeeding at all, start again at hourly intervals at the hour and work up again. Try not to make the intervals less than an hour, if at all possible; if you really have to, do so only at "peak production periods".

(d) If you are being successful, continue steadily adding a quarter of an hour to your times, but be sure to stay at each level for at least a week before trying the next.

(e) Some people find that a regular time pattern is a better discipline. If you prefer this system, work up until you can regularly hold on for about two hours. When you do this you should try to find a pattern. Only if no pattern of any kind emerges from your original three-day test (page 22) should you stick to a rigid pattern of two hours or more.

(f) When you can hold on for two to three hours, stop keeping a record unless the trouble recurs. If it does, go back to intervals half an hour shorter than your frequency and work up gradually again.

(g) When you finally feel secure, try to forget about the system as far as you can.

Those people whose incontinence shows a pattern of time or quantity, but with quite long, or very variable, intervals.

Make out Chart 2, filling in the left-hand column with your pattern of time or quantity transferred from your Pattern Chart 1.

(a)   Then fill in your new Pattern B times half an hour *before* your regular pattern times or your times of maximum production.

(b)   Go to the toilet at exactly the times on the chart.

(c)   If you are not successful, shorten the interval by a quarter of an hour until you are.

(d)   Record these times for six weeks at least, adjusting until you succeed, by which time you or your helpers will know the pattern.

(e)   If in spite of the pattern you are periodically incontinent, or need the toilet at inconvenient times, look again at your fluid intake chart and experiment to see if altering amounts or times of drinks will help.

(f)   Note carefully from your Chart 1 how long after a drink you need the toilet so that, if you need to be dry for a longer period than usual, you can adjust the time of your drink accordingly.

GROUP C

People who have no pattern of urine production.

Make out a Chart 1 and see at what times you have been urinating, even without a pattern. Go to the toilet half an hour earlier than the times on the previous day, and see if this helps over a period of a few days. Make sure your bladder is as empty as possible (see page 40). Record the results for one week on Chart 2, as for Group A2.

If there is no change, make out a Chart 2 with a pattern of 1½ hour regular intervals. Go to the toilet at these times *and at no other.* Record the results over one week, and then depending on the results, you can either extend or reduce the interval by a quarter of an hour, but not reducing to less than an hour. When you have maintained this pattern for a week, extend the periods by a quarter of an hour, staying at each level for at least a week or for as long as it takes you to feel comfortable. Don't try to extend the intervals too far and *do* keep to a very regular routine.

CHART 2 – PRESENT PATTERN TAKEN FROM ASSESSMENT OF CHART 1

Group	Time	Present Pattern	New Pattern	1	2	3	4	5	6	7	8	9	10
A1, C & D	8.45	√2cX	√	X2c	X2c	X2c	√2c	√2c	√2c	X2c	√2c	√2c	X2c
	9.00												
	9.15	√2c/1c											
	9.30												
	9.45	√½c		X2c	D2c	X2c	√2c	X2c	√2c	√2c	√2c	√2c	√2c
	10.00		√										
	10.15	√1c											
	10.30					D2c	√2c	D2c					
	10.45	√1cX						X2c	√2c	√2c	√2c	√2c	√2c
	11.00		√										
	11.15	√1c											

and so on, throughout the day . . .

Group	Time	Present Pattern	New Pattern
A2	9.00	√2cX	√
	9.15	↑	↑
	9.30	↓ ¾ hr	1 hr
	9.45	√1c(X√)	↓
	10.00	↑	√
	10.15	1 hr	↑
	10.30	↓	1¼ hr
	10.45	√1c(X√)	↓
	11.00	↑	
	11.15	1 hr	√
	11.30	↓	↑
	11.45	√1c√	
	12.00		1¼ hr
	12.15		
	12.30		√
	12.45		
	1.00		

and so on, throughout the day . . .

Group	Time	Present Pattern	New Pattern
B	9.00	√2cX	√
	9.30	√2cX	√
	10.00		
	10.30		
	11.00		√ between
	11.30		√ these two
	12.00	√1cX	
	12.30		√
	1.00	√1c√	
	1.30		
	2.00		
	2.30		√ between
	3.00		√ these two
	3.30	√1cX	
	4.00		

and so on, throughout the day . . .

c = cup(s) √ = go to toilet D = dry, but before time X = wet

People with persistent dribbling.

If you have persistent dribbling, do make sure your doctor has *all* the facts; he will want to be sure that pressure on your system has been reduced to a minimum. He may suggest the occasional use of a catheter; this is not discussed here, as it is a matter requiring professional advice.

You can help yourself by making sure that you empty your bladder as completely as possible every time you go to the toilet, as explained on page 40. Do be extra persistent in doing your pelvic floor exercises, concentrating particularly on the *feel* of stopping and starting, so that you are more aware of a dribble and can positively try to stop the flow by contracting, as in your exercises. Your stomach muscles are also very important, as they help you to expel urine.

Make out a Chart 2, as for Group A1 but with hourly intervals, and go to the toilet every hour at the hour, whether you want to or not, *and not in between.*

Think of your pelvic floor as soon as you are aware of dribbling; sit on a foot or folded towel to help you feel and support it.

Record your results and continue in this way for a week.

At the end of the week review these results. If you have not been entirely successful, continue for another week, or until you feel confident enough to extend the times by a quarter of an hour. Repeat by the week as you make progress, but don't try for too much.

For you, general exercises are important, as they will strengthen your muscles and increase your awareness of your body.

FAECAL INCONTINENCE

Faecal incontinence may be caused by many things, but it is a symptom that something is wrong with the lower digestive system. People vary greatly in their habits, from three stools a day to one every three or four days; if your normal pattern alters appreciably for more than a few days, you should see your doctor.

Faecal incontinence is a most distressing affliction, causing suffering to both patients and helpers; however, much can be done to cure, alleviate or control the condition.

Three main parts of the lower digestive system may suffer damage:

The pelvic floor, which supports the bowel and rectum.

The muscles controlling the outlet of the rectum and anus.

Sensation and function, because of interruption of nerve pathways to the brain and spinal cord.

Any of these may cause malfunction of the *mechanisms* of continence sufficient to result in leakage. A major factor in this is the strength and tone of the pelvic floor muscles. Normally the tension in the pelvic floor maintains a kink between the rectum and the anus, as seen below in diagram A. This stops faeces from escaping. When the urge to defecate arrives, the pelvic floor muscles relax, and the kink is lost, allowing faeces to be expelled (see diagram B). However, when the pelvic floor muscles are weak or damaged and sag, the situation remains permanently as in diagram B, and so continence is lost. Malfunction *within* the bowels and rectum, for whatever reason, causes either diarrhoea or constipation, often severe. When the mechanisms of continence are not working properly, the likelihood of incontinence caused by diarrhoea or constipation is increased. Other factors can seriously affect continence, such as lack of mobility or uncongenial environment: lack of privacy, having to use bedpans, cold or dirty lavatories and so on.

Causes of damage to the mechanisms of continence and some possible treatments

NERVE PATHWAY INTERRUPTION

Causes	Stroke, spinal injury, Parkinson's disease, dementia, diabetes, multiple sclerosis and others.
Treatment	Control of the consistency of the stool with planned use of constipating agents, followed by planned evacuation of the bowel. A diet to suit the individual and an attempt to find a pattern of defecation, or, when there is no sensation, looking for signs such as rapid heart rate or sweating before bowel movement. Where there is no sensation at all, some doctors may suggest colostomy.

DAMAGE TO SPHINCTERS

Cause	Loss of reflex inhibition, due to a constantly distended

bowel, straining at stool, haemorrhoids, anal fissure or prolapse of rectum.

Treatment   Appropriate diet, local treatments, surgery.

There is now a new operation to create a replacement sphincter of the rectum.

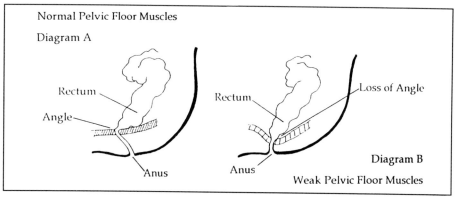

How weak pelvic floor muscles affect faecal incontinence.

DAMAGE TO PELVIC FLOOR

Causes   Years of straining at stool, chronic distension of colon, chronic constipation, birth injury, surgical injury, accident, debility and age.

Treatment   Pelvic floor exercises, Functional Electrical Stimulation, Interferential Therapy, surgery, a diet to suit the individual.

Causes of malfunction within the bowel and rectum, and some possible treatments.

DIARRHOEA

Cause   Infections or excess of food and drink.

Treatment   24 hours on water only. There may be vomiting and rumbly pain as well as diarrhoea. If it persists, see your doctor.

Cause   Ulcerative colitis.

Treatment   Doctors use antispasmodics and specialised drugs. Appropriate diet, and sometimes surgery, may be necessary.

Cause	Laxative abuse.
Treatment	Control of diet, using fibre and bulking agents rather than harsh laxatives. Suppositories may be used if there is bowel damage.
Cause	Tumours.
Treatment	Appropriate diet, specialised drugs and perhaps surgery.
Cause	Antibiotics, iron tonics and other drugs.
Treatment	Appropriate diet and change of drugs.

Chalk and opium mixtures, as well as a low-fibre diet, are used to control consistency of stool.

IRRITABLE BOWEL SYNDROME.

Causes	Unknown. Symptoms are intermittent pain and wind, with diarrhoea of no known origin.
Treatment	Doctors use peppermint oil, preferably in a capsule with paste, which coats the whole bowel in order to combat wind and pain.

CONSTIPATION

Causes	Low residue diet, low liquid diet (often from fear of urinary incontinence) and uncongenial environment, as mentioned earlier.
Treatment	High fibre and higher liquid diet. Lactulose, artificial bulk-makers and stool-softening agents.
Cause	Slower passage of food through gut. As the body ages, the pace at which food passes through the bowel slows down, largely as a result of reduced mobility. Idiopathic megacolon, irritable bowel syndrome, diverticulitis and diminished nerve supply also can have this effect.
Treatment	Change of diet and more liquid, use of lactulose and bulk-producers; liquid paraffin is sometimes used.
Cause	Psychiatric problems: depression, anxiety, confusion, anorexia and bowel phobia.

Treatment	Psychiatric help, understanding care and moral support are the most effective.
Cause	Pathological problems: diabetes, hypothyroidism and tumours can all cause constipation.
Treatment	That required for the disease, with help from diet: lactulose and bulk producers, the same as for local difficulties such as piles and anal fissures.
Cause	Drugs: some drugs, such as analgesics and those used to treat Parkinson's disease, can cause constipation.
Treatment	Change of drugs and use of non-irritant laxatives may help.

FAECAL IMPACTION

When the contents of the bowel stay too long in the colon and rectum, water is extracted to such an extent that the stool becomes very hard and gets stuck in the rectum. The result is that faecal material builds up, allowing bacteria to flourish, and irritation occurs.

A foul-smelling liquid then seeps round the rocky stool, and the muscle of the anus cannot contain the matter. This is, of course, an extreme case, but any hard stool causes straining, which may damage the pelvic floor and lead the sufferer to take irritant laxatives.

This condition is treated over a period of seven to ten days by small modern enemas, until the rectum and lower colon are truly empty. Great care must then be taken to regulate the bowels; suppositories and an occasional enema may still be necessary.

GENERAL POINTS ON FAECAL INCONTINENCE

Disposable pads or garments are best, and wingfold pads in net pants seem to be the most acceptable. Changing as soon as possible after soiling, and the use of odour-controlling products, are essential; disposal must be into airtight bags.

Washing is obviously important for both patients and helpers. Portable air-changing units, with filters which absorb the odour rather than merely masking it, are now available. Modern commodes are much better designed than the older models.

DISPOSABLE GARMENTS

STICKY-BACKED SANITARY TOWELS

suitable for   very light, and light incontinence

special feature   available in various degrees of absorbency and so suitable for a range of incontinence, when ease of buying and appearance of normality are considered of most importance; they are no use to men, as they slip even when stuck on; not made to absorb the quantity of urine which even light incontinence produces, and not always secure. A new generation of towels have one-way-wet outer skin and incorporate super-absorbent gel granules, which add greatly to absorbency and a prolonged dry feel; this has made these towels of more use to the lightly incontinent.

cost   comparatively high

ease of use   easy to put on, but messy to take off if overloaded

comfort   good until quite wet, when either they move as the sticky back fails, or they break up and leak; also they fall away from the body when heavy with urine. I recommend change to superabsorbent special towels, made in various sizes, available at large chemists or from the address given at the back of the book.

SUPERABSORBENT PADS

Almost all disposable pads and garments are now made of superabsorbent material, with a waterproof backing and faced with one-way-wet material, for the feel of dryness and the protection of skin.

STICKY-BACKED INCONTINENCE PADS

suitable for   light and medium incontinence, with ordinary or special pants

special feature   better than sanitary towels, as they are specially made for urine and so much more absorbent; the sticky back lasts longer; although flat, they are larger and so

	absorb over a larger area; for men they stay in place better
cost	less than sanitary towels
ease of use	easy to put on, can be messy to take off if left too long
comfort	they may seem bulky when dry, but are much more comfortable than sanitary towels when wet; they are more secure and don't hang away from the body so much or break up so soon.

PENILE POUCHES

suitable for	light to medium incontinence
special feature	better for men than stick-on pads, can be super-absorbent
cost	medium
ease of use	easy to carry, need plastic bag for disposal when out, but quite small
comfort	fair, better than pads.

NON-STICK DISPOSABLE PADS

1. LIGHTWEIGHT SINGLE

suitable for	light and medium incontinence, used with:
	(a) external pouch in reusable pants,
	(b) internal pouch in reusable pants,
	(c) stretchable net pants
	(d) doublet and front-opening pants
special feature	mainly used for long-term incontinence, very secure; the pads are disposable – pants can be washed
cost	low
ease of use	easy to insert in pants before they are put on, but less easy to insert while pants are worn; it is a bit messy to take wet pad out while pants are worn – better to take pants off; with stretchable pants the pad is put next to the body and then pants are pulled up; they are quite easy to put on and fairly easy to take out, as pants can be slid down a little and the pad replaced. Front-opening and doublet pants are dealt with in the section on pants
comfort	depends largely on the quality and fit of the pants and pads; ideally, wash pants with every change of

pad; experiment with various makes until you find what suits you best.

2. STANDARD AND DOUBLE PADS

suitable for	medium to heavy incontinence
special feature	the same as for lightweight pads
cost	reasonable, but increases with degree of absorbency
ease of use	see comments for lightweight pads, with increased emphasis
comfort	inevitably bulkier and heavier when wet, so they tend to hang away from the body.

3. WINGFOLD PADS

suitable for	cases of heavy urinary, and also faecal, incontinence
special feature	use with net or doublet pants
cost	reasonable
ease of use	easier to use than pads with pouch; put the pad in place against the body, pull up the pants and *then* pull out the wings of the pad; do not try to open the wings until the pants are in place
comfort	the wide wings and netting hold the pad close to the body and keep the pad in shape; the large surface area spreads the weight and contains urine well.

4. SHAPED PADS

suitable for	all ages and degrees of incontinence.
special feature	are colour coded for size and absorbency
cost	fairly reasonable, usually on prescription
ease of use	are used inside net pants
comfort	all super-absorbent, but can be difficult to put on for the elderly and obese.

DISPOSABLE ALL-IN-ONE GARMENTS

1. PANTY-TYPE

suitable for	medium incontinence (see *Kimberley-Clark Ltd*, page 85)
special feature	useful for special occasions, such as outings, or when washing is difficult; also, they are practical and neat

	for everyday use if you can afford them
cost	quite expensive
ease of use	very convenient, they can be put on and taken off just like pants; some have side-buttons and elastic, so that they can be put on as a pad and then fastened; taking them off is not messy, as all liquid is contained in the pad, which is then discarded – no washing required
comfort	quite bulky when dry, but they are comfortable and remain so until very wet; they are very secure, bulky to dispose of, but otherwise easily managed.

2. FULL GARMENTS

suitable for	heavy incontinence
special feature	their very large area means that wetness is spread and contained; leg fittings mean that there is little danger of leaking
cost	expensive
ease of use	easy for the badly disabled to put on when lying down, less easy to put on when standing, but all right once you have the knack – very useful for special occasions, going out etc.
comfort	they last quite a time and are surprisingly comfortable, even when quite wet.

It is a good idea to keep a pack of these in reserve for special occasions or when washing is difficult – or indeed for regular use if you can afford them! There are many different makes of all these products; you can get advice about the right ones for you from your continence adviser or from centres such as the Dene Centre, which has a room full of samples and an advisory and helpline service (address at the back of the book).

REUSABLE GARMENTS, PADS AND BEDDING

PANTS WITH BUILT-IN PADS

suitable for	light and light-medium incontinence
special feature	they look like normal briefs or Y-fronts with opening
cost	about half as much again as cotton briefs and Y-fronts
ease of comfort	very comfortable, one-way-wet lining keeps you

feeling dry, and the backing stops leaks; remains close to the body, and there is no smell; they are very secure; wash as ordinary pants at up to 60°F, but do not use bleach or fabric softener; a powder such as *Bold* is satisfactory.

I especially recommend these garments for almost everybody who is independent or who has access to even ordinary washing facilities.

1. Pants made of one-way-wet fabric with a "marsupial" pouch which holds a disposable pad. There are male and female styles.

2. Lightweight washable elasticated mesh pants which hold a pad securely in place.

3. Superabsorbent pad made of one-way-wet fabric with an adhesive strip.

4. & 5. A disposable penile pouch with waterproof backing and super-absorbent lining; it can be held in place by close-fitting under-wear, shown in 5.

6. A complete, all-in-one disposable garment suitable for heavy incontinence.

7. A disposable panty-type garment for medium incontinence.

8. A shaped pad available in all sizes and absorbencies, colour coded for size and absorbency, worn under net pants.

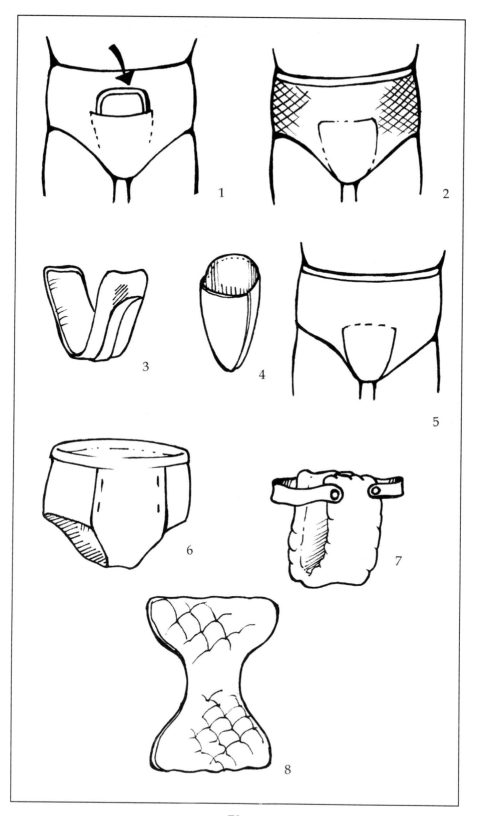

POUCH PANTS WITH OUTSIDE OR INSIDE POUCH

suitable for   all degrees of incontinence, with varying sizes of pad and degrees of absorbency

special features   the different makes of pants vary, but most are knitted fabric and made for either sex; you can choose an inside or outside pouch; inside pouches are a little more difficult to load and unload, but the pad is held close to you by the whole garment, and some people feel that this is less conspicuous; outside pouches can be made with Y-front opening; these pants last for about a year

cost   reasonable

ease of use   see comments in section on pads

comfort   depends on the fit and the make and type of pad; find those that suit you best.

NET PANTS

suitable for   all degrees of incontinence

special features   reusable a few times and very versatile; they are compact to carry, can be washed under a tap and dry quickly

cost   cheap per item, so reasonable over a period

ease of use   easy for all but the very disabled

comfort   very comfortable, provided they are the right size, as they keep pads very secure; make sure they have two-way stretch, side to side and up and down.
I recommend these.

FRONT-OPENING AND DOUBLET POUCH PANTS

suitable for   all degrees of incontinence

special feature   excellent for the physically handicapped

cost   a little more expensive than the normal pouch, but they last for about a year

ease of use   *Velcro* and press studs make them usable by all but the most severely disabled, and so help to keep you independent

comfort   as for normal pouch pants.

74

WATERPROOF PANTS

suitable for	light and medium incontinence
special feature	you can now buy waterproof pants that allow the air to get in and don't rustle
cost	reasonable
ease of use	as for normal pants
comfort	they are very secure, but their efficiency depends on the pad or pants and pad worn underneath them; they tend to harden with washing and do not last very long.

PENILE SHEATHS

These are special condom-like sheaths with a sticky strip for attachment, connected to a collecting bag which is removable for emptying and is attached to the leg in a holster inside the trousers. For many men with heavy to severe incontinence these sheaths and bags are invaluable. There are now special sheaths available for short and retracted penises.

MALE URINALS

These are collecting bottles and should have a top or a non-spill device. There are both reusable and disposable varieties available from chemists or from the addresses at the back of the book.

FEMALE URINALS

They can be made of metal or plastic, with a disposable collector. The best ones are shaped to the female form and can be used without the collector, for travelling, as they hold a certain amount on their own. A plastic funnel attached to a tube leading to any receptacle can be a useful home-made urinal and can be used almost anywhere. The collection bags are available on the NHS, but urinals have to be paid for. The address is given at the back of the book.

DISPOSABLE BEDDING AND FURNITURE PROTECTORS

BED AND CHAIR SQUARES

These are made of cellulose, with waterproof backing, and will keep a bed or chair dry for two to three hours. They can also be used for padding round patients in bed. Their disadvantage is that they tend to move, becoming crumpled and so uncomfortable.

SHEETS AND PILLOWCASES

These are available from most big chemists and are useful when you are away from home or when laundry is difficult (other addresses are at the back of the book).

REUSABLE BEDDING AND FURNITURE COVERS

WATERPROOF BEDCOVERS

A wide range of fitted and unfitted mattress and pillow covers are available from chemists and through the National Health Service, and also through the Mail Order Service. Tuck-in bed protectors are available, as well as full bedcovers. There are other addresses at the back of the book for washable, waterproof duvet-covers and blanket-protectors, which are particularly useful for men.

Points to look out for

1. See that the quality is good enough; every person incontinent in bed will need at least two of these items. As they will require constant wiping and washing, they must stand up to hard wear.
2. The material must allow for the passage of air, so that the old problems of sweat and condensation are avoided.
3. The surface must not wrinkle when anchored.
4. They must protect a large enough area, so that you do not spoil mattresses.
5. Make sure that both you and your washing and drying arrangements can manage the bulk and the weight of the cover. I suggest *Kylie*, or similar, bed protectors for most users, as they are lightweight and easy to manage, and meet the other requirements.
   They can be used over a full mattress cover if required; in this way the bulky item need not be washed so frequently.
6. Costs vary; look out for good buys, bearing in mind the points above.

ORDINARY SHEETS

Easy-care sheets are ideal, with as large a percentage of cotton as possible, both for comfort and for hygiene. Nylon is not suitable, and anything that needs ironing should be avoided, unless you have unlimited help. Pretty or colourful sheets make you feel less of an invalid and cheer you up.

PADDED SQUARES, BEDSHEETS AND CHAIR COVERS

These are readily available, but they vary considerably in price and quality. A cotton cover on a square can be used for outings. Ask for advice if you are not sure what you need.

Points to look out for

1. With a bedsheet, make sure that the padded area is large enough.
2. The absorbency must not be so great that you cannot cope with the wet article.
3. The surface must breathe and not wrinkle; it must be soft enough for comfort.
4. Make sure that there is no danger of plastic burn from the underlying bed-protector.
5. With chair covers, make sure that the protective surface comes a little way up the sides of the chair.
6. Make sure that chair squares are large enough.
7. The padded covers should be washable in an ordinary hot wash, up to 95°F.
8. Look out for special instructions, such as avoiding bleach or fabric softeners.

One-way-wet bedsheets and chair covers are made of soft one-way-wet top layer with an absorbent layer attached below; this is anchored by side tuck-ins that stop the sheet from wrinkling. A bed-protector or waterproof mattress cover is placed under the sheet.

There are two versions of the sheet available:

(a) **standard** – holding up to 3 litres of urine,
(b) **lightweight** – holding up to 1½ litres.

The lightweight sheet is sufficient for most uses and is much easier to handle when wet and to wash than the standard.

The patient stays dry, and *there is no need for pads of any kind.* Top-only or back-opening nightwear should be used, as the greater the area of skin in contact with the sheet the better it will work.

This arrangement allows the whole skin area to breathe and the sufferer to feel normal, and there is only the sheet to wash. It takes courage to put yourself with no pad into a bed that you know will be wet, but – **have courage!** You will be dry, comfortable and unfettered.

The sheet can be washed as normal cotton, up to 60°F, but do not add bleach or fabric-softener. It is guaranteed for up to 200 washes, but when washed at home it lasts for many more; in fact the more it is washed the softer and thicker it becomes. It is not suitable for faecal incontinence.

You will need two sheets, one on and one off; a bedridden person will need three. This means quite a large initial outlay, but you do not need to buy pants or pads, so over a period these sheets are economical. They *really* combat soreness and increase comfort and dignity. **I strongly recommend them.**

The chair-covers can be used as normal covers with a waterproof under-cover; they can also be used in the same way as the bedsheet, with back-opening clothes and no pants or pads, without attracting any attention.

Makers and suppliers are listed at the end of the book.

Local numbers (for you to fill in):

Doctor ....

Continence Adviser ....

District Nurse ....

District Hospital ....

District Day Hospital ....

Social Worker ....

Physiotherapist ....

Occupational Therapist ....

Unit where pads and pants are collected ....

Meals on Wheels ....

Department of Social Security ....

Department of Health ....

Department of Social Services ....

W.R.V.S. ....

Disabled Drivers' Association ....

Dial-A-Ride ....

Church ....

Trade Union ....

Business Personnel Officer ....

Others: ....

....

....

....

....

....

Local Red Cross* ....

Citizens' Advice Bureau* ....

* These two organisations are particularly useful. The Red Cross will lend or lease wheelchairs, commodes, etc. and will provide help with transport, meals and many other things. The Citizens' Advice Bureau is a mine of helpful information. The people who work there are extremely knowledgeable and can be consulted on a very wide range of subjects.

Age Concern, Astral House, 1268 London Rd, Norbury, SW16 4ER. Tel 081-679 8000 – *special advice for the elderly and those who care for them.*

The Association for Continence Advice, The Basement, Doughty St, WC1N 2PH. Tel 071-404 6821.

The Association of Crossroads Care Attendance Schemes, 10 Regent's Place, Rugby, Warks. Tel (0788) 573653 – *relief care attendants scheme.*

The Association of Retired Persons – ARP – 20/30 Fitzroy Sq, London WE1P 5HH. Tel 071-895 8880 – *consumer association for the over-fifties, with legal, community and help advice.*

The Association of Spina Bifida and Hydrocephalus, 56 Camberwell Rd, London SE5. Tel 071-252 6325.

The Association to aid Sexual and Personal Relationships for People with a Disability – SPOD – 286 Camden Rd, London N7 0BJ. Tel 071-607 8851.

The Alzheimer's Disease Society, Gordon House, 10 Greencoats Place, London SW1P 1PH. Tel 071-306 0606 – *monthly newsletter, local support groups, open learning for carers.*

The British Diabetic Association, 10 Queen Anne St, London W1. Tel 071-323 1531.

The British Epilepsy Association, Anstey House, 40 Hanover Sq, Leeds LS3 1BE. Tel (0532) 439393.

The Carers' National Association, 29 Chilworth Mews, London W2 3RG. Tel 071-724 7776 – *will give help and information, including nearest local help.*

The Continence Foundation, The Basement, 2 Doughty St, London WC1N 2PH – *newly established foundation to co-ordinate activities in promotion of continence.*

The Dene Centre, Castle's Farm Road, Newcastle upon Tyne NE3 1PH. Tel 091-284 0480 – *gives comprehensive help for the disabled, with a unit for incontinence which includes expert medical advice, a room full of garments and pads, with an adviser at hand to help with these and with toilet and clothing difficulties, also a personal helpline which can be used by people from all over Britain.*

The Disabled Living Foundation, 380-384 Harrow Rd, London W9 2HU. Tel 071-289 6111 – *permanent exhibition of aids, books, tapes etc, but one must make an appointment.*

The Disablement Income Group – DIG – Mill Mead Business Centre, Mill Mead Rd, London N17 9QU. Tel 081-801 8013 – *advice and information on finances and quarterly newsletter 'DIG Around'.*

The Enuresis Resource and Information Centre – ERIC – 65 St Michael's Hill, Bristol BS2 8DZ. Tel (0272) 264 920 – *all help for bedwetters.*

Help for Health, Highcroft Cottage, Romsey Rd, Winchester SO22 5DH. Tel (0345) 678 679 – *information line and quarterly newsletter which is free in Wessex and £5 outside.*

The Glasgow Continence Resource Centre – Southern General Hospital, Glasgow G51 4TF. Tel 041 445 2455 ext 3352 or 3444.

Help the Aged, St James's Walk, London EC1R. Tel 071-253 0253.

IBS Network (Irritable Bowel Syndrome), c/o Wells Park Health Project, 1A Wells Park Rd, Sydenham, London SE26 6JE – *help for bowel problems with newsletter 'Gut Reaction'.*

Incontact, (National Action on Incontinence), 4 St Pancras Way, London NW1 0PE – *consumers' association and support group.*

The International Continence Society, Southmead Hospital, Bristol BS10 5NB. Tel (0272) 505 050. Department of Urology, Dr P. Abrams.

The Invalid Children's Aid Association, 3 Keith Grove, London W12. Tel 081-749 1681.

MIND, 22 Harley St, London W1N 2ED. Tel 071- 637 0741.

The MS Society, 25 Effie Rd, London SW6 1EE. Tel 071-736 6267.

The Patients' Association, 18 Victoria Park Sq, London E2 9PF. Tel 081-981 5676.

The Royal Association for Disability and Rehabilitation – RADAR – 25 Mortimer St, London W1N 8AB. Tel 071-637 5400 – *information of all kinds and a monthly bulletin (see Magazines).*

The Royal Society for Mentally Handicapped Children, 123 Golden Lane, London EC1Y 0RT. Tel 071-636 5020.

The Spastics Society, 12 Park Crescent, London W1N 4EQ. Tel 071-636 5052.

The Spinal Injuries Association, Yeoman's House, St James's Lane, London N10. Tel 081- 444 2121.

Across Trust (Jumbulance), Bridge House, East Molesey, Surrey KT8 9HF. Tel 081-783 1355 – _fully adapted coach with trained medical staff, for holidays and pilgrimages abroad._

Care Match, 286 Camden Rd, London N7 0PJ. Tel 071-609 9966 – _computer matching of homes for physically disabled people._

Care Search, Fairways, St Briavel's, Lydney, Glos. Tel (0594) 530 220 – _home finding by computer._

Crossroads Care Attendant Trust, 10 Regent's Place, Rugby, Warks. Tel (0788) 73653.

Elderly Accommodation Counsel, 46A Chiswick High Rd, London W4 1SZ. Tel 081-742 1182 or 081-995 8320 – _national computer-based information on nursing homes, residential homes and sheltered accommodation._

GRACE Care Home Advice, 35 Walnut Tree Close, Guildford, Surrey. Tel (0483) 304354.

Home Farm Trust, Merchant House, North Wapping Road, Bristol BS1 4RW. Tel (0272) 273746.

John Routledge Hunter Memorial Fund – Mr. Norman Robson, c/o Dickinson, Miller Turnbull, Cross House, Westgate Road, Newcastle 1. Tel 091-261 1911 – 10.30 to noon, Thursdays -_holidays for people from Newcastle and Northumberland._

The Leonard Cheshire Foundation, 26 Maunsell Street, London SW1. Tel 071-828 1822.

Mencap Homes Foundation, 123 Golden Road, London EC1Y 0RT. Tel 071-454 0454.

MIND, 22 Harley Street, London W1N 2ED. Tel 071-262 1451.

The Star Centre, Urchinwood Manor, Cheltenham, Glos.

Tel (0242) 527631 – _a residential centre for training handicapped students._

RADAR, 25 Mortimer St, London W1N 8AB. Tel 071-637 5400 – _information on holidays at home and worldwide._

Adult Bedwetters and their Problems.	Harry Stone	The Cyrenians Ltd, 13 Wincheap, Canterbury, Kent.
Be Confident, Be Continent	The MS Society	25 Effie Road, London SW6 1EE
Childhood Incontinence	Roger Morgan BA, PhD	Disabled Living Foundation or Heinemann Medical Books, 23 Bedford Square, WC1B 3HH
Coping and Caring – A Guide to Identifying and Supporting an Elderly Person with Dementia (a very useful guide)	Dr Brian Lodge	Mind, 155/157 Woodhouse Lane, Leeds LS2 2EF
Coping with Ageing Parents	C.G. Gilhead & G.Watt	Macdonald Ltd, Loanhead, Midlothian, Scotland.
Forgetfulness in the Elderly – Advice for Carers	Age Concern	Astral House, 1268 London Rd, Norbury, SW16 4ER
Health Directory (lists 1,000 agencies to help patients and families)		Harper & Row Ltd, Estover Road, Plymouth. PL6 7PZ.
Incontinence	Dorothy Mandelstam	Disabled Living Foundation, or Heinemann, addresses above
A New Deal for Carers		The King's Fund Centre, 126 Albert St, London NW1 7NF. £4.50 incl. p&p.

Caring at Home		As above
Sexual and Personal Relationships of the Disabled		SPOD, 286 Camden Road, London N7 0BJ
24-Hour Approach to Problems of Confusion	Una Holden and others	Winslow Press, 23 Horn Street, Winslow, Bucks. MK18 3AP
Who Cares? (very helpful on all fronts)	Dr J. Miller	BBC Education, Room 202, Villiers House, London W5 2PA
Constipation, Piles and other Bowel Disorders.	R. Heatley	Churchill Livingstone
The Irritable Bowel book	Rosemary Nicol	Sheldon Press, £3.50
Toilet Training and Bed-wetting, a Practical Guide	Heather Welford	Thomson's publishing £2.99

BEDPANS, URINALS, COMMODES, DEODORANTS, PADS, PANTS AND BEDDING

DISPOSABLE PADS AND GARMENTS

There is a great range of disposable garments available; those included here all have something special to recommend them, and it is worth finding out what suits you best. All are superabsorbent.

Coloplast Ltd, Peterborough Business Park, Peterborough, PE2 OFX *Conveen range of stick-on towels, fact sheet, help line, Ostobon.* Mail Order Freephone 0800 622 124

LIC Care Ltd, B11, Armstrong Mall, Southwood, Farnborough, GU14 ONR *Daisy range of pads and garments with unique anti-bacterial agent that protects skin and combats odour.*

Procter and Gamble, PO Box 1EE, Newcastle upon Tyne, NE99 1EE *Attends Ultra range of midi self-adhesive pads, maxi pads held in net pants, full garments. Freephone 0800 590555.*

Robinson Healthcare, Hipper House, Chesterfield, S40 1YF *Inco-care full range of pads and garments including wingfold and waterproof pants, chair and bed pads and multipurpose wipes.*

Kimberley-Clark Ltd, Larkfield, Aylesford, Kent, ME20 7PS *Depend self-adhesive pads, unique bikini and fitted brief, advisory service, freephone for ordering 0800 521 128*

REUSABLE PADS AND GARMENTS

Ganmill Ltd, 38/40 Market Street, Bridgwater, Somerset TA6 3EP *Unitex range of very good waterproof backed one-way-wet cotton chair/bedcover, male/female butterfly pad and pants. Also see under commodes, telephone 0278 423037*

Anglia Vale Medical Ltd, Unit 6, Lancaster Way Business Complex, Ely, OB6 3NW *Wide range including terry shaped and straight pads with waterproof backing.*

Wellcross Healthcare Ltd, 2 Wellcross, Edith Weston, Rutland, LE15 8HG *Carewell full range including whole garment with waterproof outer layer. See also under bedding section.*

Roche Products Ltd, PO Box 8, Welwyn Garden City, AL7 3AY *Kylie range of one-way-wet absorbent bed sheets, chair covers and pants. Pants very good for light incontinence.*

BEDDING

Anti-crackle, anti-sweat, washable bedding including duvets and pillows.

Feeder Products Ltd, PO Box 481, Blackmore, Ingatestone, Essex CM4 0NA

Wellcross Healthcare Ltd, see under reusable pads

Mackworth Medical Products Ltd, Bradford Street, Caerphilly, Glam. CF8 1GA

Loxley Medical Supplies, Unit 5D, Carnaby Industrial Estate, Bridlington, North Humberside. *Nilodor.*

Coloplast Ltd, see under disposable pads. *Ostobon.*

Simcare, see under sheaths and collection bags. *Chironair, Ozium.*

Thackerycare, see under sheaths and collection bags. (see De Puy Healthcare)

Cool Heat Ltd, 167 Hullbridge Road, South Woodham Ferrers, Chelmsford, Essex CM3 5LN *Portable air changer with special odour-absorbing filter.*

MMG (Europe) Ltd, Redland House, Bristol BS6 6YE. Tel (0272) 736 883 – *they supply* **Natural Odour Neutralizer** *(XO) which can be used on animals, carpets etc. It eats odours by biological action and is biodegradable – also reusable bedding and pads.*

MALE AND FEMALE URINALS, COLLECTION BAGS AND CATHETERS

Bard Ltd, Forrest House, Brighton Road, Crawley, West Sussex RH11 9BP *Catheters for all purposes including hydrogel coated and pre-filled. Unique finger grip on intermittent catheter. Collection bags with simple safe taps.*

Simcare, Peter Road, Lancing, West Sussex, BN15 8TJ *Full range of catheters, collection bags and sheaths; also Reddy Bottle disposable flat pack urinal for men.*

Hollister Ltd, 43 Castle Street, Reading, RG1 7SN *Incare male sheaths, collection bags; also female urinary pouch and faecal collector, fact sheets and help line.*

De Puy Healthcare, Millsham House, Manor Mill Lane, Leeds, LS11 8LQ. Tel (0532) 706000 *Aquadry self-adhesive penile sheaths including "aquadry plus" for retracted and short penises and collection bags with "no chafe" straps, also non-spill adaptor for urine bottle.*

Codan (UK) Ltd, Eastheath Avenue, Wokingham, RG11 2PR *Mille female urinal.* Tel (0734) 783 663

BIDETS AND COMMODES

Ganmill Ltd, see under reusable garments *Very good "Unitex" -replaces lavatory if necessary.*

Joncare, Radley Road Industrial Estate, Abingdon, OX14 3RY

Vernon Carus Ltd, Penwortham Mills, Preston, PR1 9SN *Unique disposal system for pads in the home, also disposable pads etc.*

PELVIC FLOOR STRENGTHENING

Colgate Medical Ltd, Freepost SL1669, Windsor SL4 4BR *Femina vaginal cones.*

Nidd Valley Micro Products Ltd, Thistle Hill, Knaresborough, North Yorkshire HG5 8JW *Acupad electrical therapy unit, to be used with help from physiotherapist or continence adviser. Hire service available.*

VIDEOS

Where is the Key?, Suffer the Carers, Communication in dementia and others can be hired from the Alzheimer's Disease Society -address above.

Out and About and Dry. Dr. Katherine Moore explains retraining schemes for urge incontinence. Tel 0727 840041 (Free)

HELPLINES, TELEPHONE TAPES AND ADVICE

ARMS – Action Research for MS – *advice* – 071-222 3123.

Coloplast Helpline – Freephone (0800) 622124.

CRUSE – *help and advice for the bereaved* – 081-940 4818.

The Dene Centre, now the National Helpline – *comprehensive personal advice on all aspects of urinary and faecal incontinence, including information on all makes of pads, garments and protective items* – 091-213 0050. *Monday to Friday 3 to 7 p.m.*

Dial U.K. – *information and advice on disability* – (0302) 310123.

DIG (Disabled Income Group) – 081-801 8013

Disabled Living Foundation – 071-289 6111. *Monday to Friday 10 a.m. to 3.55 p.m.*

Glasgow Continence Resource Helpline – 041 425 1117.

Health Call – *three-minute tape on incontinence* – (0898) 600835.

Help for Health – *24-hour answering service* – (0345) 678 679

Help the Aged – 0800 289 404. *Monday to Friday 10 a.m. to 4 p.m.*

Incare Helpline – Freephone (0800) 521377.

MIND – *advice 2-4.40 p.m., legal advice 2-5 p.m.* – 071-637 0741.

Multiple Sclerosis – 071-371 8000. *Monday to Friday 10 a.m. to 4 p.m.*

National Spinal Injuries – 081-883 4246. *Monday and Friday 2 to 4 p.m., Tuesday, Wednesday and Thursday 4 to 8 p.m.*

The Patients' Association – 081-981 5676.

MAGAZINES

Disability Now, 12 Park Crescent, London W1N 4EQ.

Home and Dry, Incare Ltd, 43 Castle Street, Reading RG1 7SN.

RADAR Bulletin, 11 copies annually £6.50, from RADAR, 25 Mortimer Street, London W1N 8AB.

This Caring Business, 1 St. Thomas's Street, Hastings, E. Sussex TN34 3LG.

"Can't Wait" Cards, obtainable from the MS Society, *a small card saying "because of illness which is not infectious, I need to go to the toilet urgently.*

Thank you". repeated in French, German and Spanish.

Disabled Toilet Key Scheme – keys can be bought from "RADAR", £3.75 incl. p & p, with list of all disabled toilets in the UK.

MAIL ORDER SERVICE

PADS DIRECT, Cranfield Rd, Logstock, Bolton, Lancs. Telephone orders – credit card – (0204) 668 800, or send cheque for 24-hour delivery service; a good selection of very reasonably priced, mainly disposable, pads and bedding.

KAROMED LTD, Karomed House, Millfield, Chard, Somerset. Telephone orders – credit card or cheque – (0460) 67761: as PADS DIRECT, but has a larger range of reusables and bedding, furniture and household aids of all sorts.

	Present pattern	New Pattern	Day 1 Meal or snack	Amount of drink	Urgency	Success	Amount of urine	Medicine	Day 2 Meal or snack	Amount of drink	Urgency	Success	Amount of urine	Medicine	Day 3 Meal or snack	Amount of drink	Urgency	Success	Amount of urine	Medicine
7.00 a.m.																				
7.15																				
7.30																				
7.45																				
8.00																				
8.15																				
8.30																				
8.45																				
9.00																				
9.15																				
9.30																				
9.45																				
10.00																				
10.15																				
10.30																				
10.45																				
11.00																				
11.15																				
11.30																				
11.45																				
12.00																				
12.15 p.m.																				
12.30																				
12.45																				
1.00																				
1.15																				
1.30																				
1.45																				
2.00																				
2.15																				
2.30																				
2.45																				
3.00																				
3.15																				
3.30																				
3.45																				
4.00																				
4.15																				

✓ = go   x = wet   D = get to toilet in time   x/D = sometimes wet, sometimes dry.   Amount in cups or fluid ounces.

	Present pattern	New Pattern	Day 1						Day 2						Day 3					
			Meal or snack	Amount of drink	Urgency	Success	Amount of urine	Medicine	Meal or snack	Amount of drink	Urgency	Success	Amount of urine	Medicine	Meal or snack	Amount of drink	Urgency	Success	Amount of urine	Medicine
4.30 p.m.																				
4.45																				
5.00																				
5.15																				
5.30																				
5.45																				
6.00																				
6.15																				
6.30																				
6.45																				
7.00																				
7.15																				
7.30																				
7.45																				
8.00																				
8.15																				
8.30																				
8.45																				
9.00																				
9.15																				
9.30																				
9.45																				
10.00																				
10.15																				
10.30																				
10.45																				
11.00																				
12.00																				
1.00 a.m.																				
2.00																				
3.00																				
4.00																				
5.00																				
6.00																				
7.00																				
Total drunk and passed during day																				

✓ = go   x = wet   D = get to toilet in time   x/D = sometimes wet, sometimes dry.   Amount in cups or fluid ounces.

	Present pattern	New Pattern	Meal or snack	Amount of drink	Urgency	Success	Amount of urine	Medicine	Meal or snack	Amount of drink	Urgency	Success	Amount of urine	Medicine	Meal or snack	Amount of drink	Urgency	Success	Amount of urine	Medicine
					Day 1						Day 2						Day 3			
7.00 a.m.																				
7.15																				
7.30																				
7.45																				
8.00																				
8.15																				
8.30																				
8.45																				
9.00																				
9.15																				
9.30																				
9.45																				
10.00																				
10.15																				
10.30																				
10.45																				
11.00																				
11.15																				
11.30																				
11.45																				
12.00																				
12.15 p.m.																				
12.30																				
12.45																				
1.00																				
1.15																				
1.30																				
1.45																				
2.00																				
2.15																				
2.30																				
2.45																				
3.00																				
3.15																				
3.30																				
3.45																				
4.00																				
4.15																				

✓ = go   x = wet   D = get to toilet in time   x/D = sometimes wet, sometimes dry.   Amount in cups or fluid ounces.

			Day 1						Day 2						Day 3					
	Present pattern	New Pattern	Meal or snack	Amount of drink	Urgency	Success	Amount of urine	Medicine	Meal or snack	Amount of drink	Urgency	Success	Amount of urine	Medicine	Meal or snack	Amount of drink	Urgency	Success	Amount of urine	Medicine
4.30 p.m.																				
4.45																				
5.00																				
5.15																				
5.30																				
5.45																				
6.00																				
6.15																				
6.30																				
6.45																				
7.00																				
7.15																				
7.30																				
7.45																				
8.00																				
8.15																				
8.30																				
8.45																				
9.00																				
9.15																				
9.30																				
9.45																				
10.00																				
10.15																				
10.30																				
10.45																				
11.00																				
12.00																				
1.00 a.m.																				
2.00																				
3.00																				
4.00																				
5.00																				
6.00																				
7.00																				
Total drunk and passed during day																				

✓ = go   x = wet   D = get to toilet in time   x/D = sometimes wet, sometimes dry.   Amount in cups or fluid ounces.

93

"All the information that anybody wants is in [this] book and it is an excellent reference work for nurses or doctors, or indeed patients and their carers.

Prof. C.M. Castleden,
Department of Medicine for the Elderly,Leicester.

"This is a very useful little book aimed at patients with urinary incontinence and their carers, although I suspect that many doctors would also profit from reading it . . . Quite simply the book suggests that there is always something that can be done for the incontinent patient and it spells out exactly what can be achieved."

A.J. Tulloch British Journal of General Practice, August 1990.

Produced with the support of Farmitalia Carlo Erba Limited